SEIZURE

Books by Charles L. Mee, Jr.

White Robe, Black Robe
Meeting at Potsdam
A Visit to Haldeman and Other States of Mind
Seizure

Charles L. Mee, Jr.

SEIZURE

M. Evans and Company, Inc.   New York, N.Y. 10017

M. Evans and Company titles are distributed in the United States by the J. B. Lippincott Company, East Washington Square, Philadelphia, Pa. 19105; and in Canada by McClelland & Stewart Ltd., 25 Hollinger Road, Toronto M4B 3G2, Ontario.

Library of Congress Cataloging in Publication Data
Mee, Charles L
  Seizure.
    1. Brain—Tumors—Biography. 2. Morris, Kathy.
  I. Title.
RC280.B7M43   616.9'93'810926 [B]   77-26884
ISBN 0-87131-254-9

Design by Al Cetta

Manufactured in the United States of America

9 8 7 6 5 4 3 2 1

Foreword

The beginning of this story—of a young woman abruptly stricken with seizures—was told to me by a friend, a neurosurgeon. The story fascinated me at first because it was, as he told it, a history composed entirely of thoughts, impressions, and passions. Even the facts of neurology turned out to be perishing phenomena, figments of imagination. For that curious reason—and then more urgently because I just wanted to know what was going to happen—I was drawn into the story.

In these pages, I have set down the narrative as faithfully as I could, recording what I was told, and recounting what I saw. I have changed a few of the names—medical ethics preclude the use of the neurosurgeon's real name—but the patient's name and most of the other names are not altered. I have otherwise tried to tell as exactly as possible a story that is, ultimately, a mystery.

PART ONE

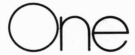

One

She thought that she could last a while longer, but, even as she thought so, as she drove from her home, from her apartment in New York, on the Upper West Side near her music school, to visit her brother, as she approached the midpoint of a tunnel somewhere on the turnpike, a white-tiled tunnel, blue-striped, neon-lit, pulsating, antiseptic and nauseating, blurred along the periphery, just when she believed she would be able to last at least until the first breath of sunlight, the first breath of trees, the first breath of green—until the first breath, anyway—then, at once, she was not at all certain who it was she was going to visit, or where he was, or what his name was, nor finally even was she any longer entirely certain at all who she was.

She thought she must stop, then, before she died, or, worse, before she fell away helplessly, spun far away and lost herself. She pulled over to the side of the turnpike then, or perhaps it was later, near a toll booth, or there near the tunnel. In any case, she stopped, and sat quietly in the car, patiently, breathing gently, looking composedly at the license plates of the

passing cars, at the turnpike ahead of her, at the line of the
horizon, at the light of the sky as it turned to orange and bright
steel, to magenta, as it sometimes seems to do along that part
of the coast. She felt distant, as though she were bearing off
swiftly across the flatlands, across the marshlands, drifting
away among the gulls and down along the tidewater where the
sounds were remote and muted, soft murmurings, dim and
indistinct. She mused and lost herself among her musings, and
when next she thought to think to be aware, she was astonished
to discover that it was dark, and that she could see the stars.

It may have been then that a policeman walked up to her and
asked whether or not she was all right. She wanted to say to
him, simply, help me, but she could not discover the words
anywhere, and she said what came easily to mind. Oh, no, she
said, I'm fine. Okay. Thanks. I'm, you know, fine.

The policeman said a word or two then, nodded, and turned
away. She wanted to bring him back, and so she called out:

I'm fine, thanks.

Sometime later she found herself at a service station, trying
to use the telephone to call her brother. She had a dime, but
she could not recall her brother's telephone number. . . . She
called her uncle, who lived nearby, near her brother's college,
in this same part of the country, but he was not at home, and
she would try later but then she could no longer remember her
uncle's telephone number or his name or the state in which he
lived. She could conjure up his face without trouble; she knew
him well enough; she could envisage his wife, too, her short
brunette hair, quickness of touch, nervousness, smile, chilly
fingertips, brown eyes—but they all, all her family, remained
completely nameless.

Oh, she said, to the two young men and the young woman,
all her age, all well-scrubbed, clean and short-haired, shaved

and pressed, fiercely normal young people, could you tell me
what time it is, or even where this is, or—here she stalled for
time, talking herself back into words and numbers, keeping up
the chatter with anything that came to mind—how far is it
to where I want to go, do you know, or where I am going, and
exactly the difference between where it is and how far I want
to go or the name of my brother?

And they, these three young strangers, were, as it happened,
Jehovah's Witnesses, who cried out at once Oh God, Praise
God Hallelujah, thank the Lord for sending you to us, for we
knew that we could help—and they gathered close around her
and held her tightly, praying and calling out to God, saying the
Lord their God was a good God and a loving God and would
care for her and all His creatures, let her put her faith in Him,
praise God, Oh! praise the Lord—and she did not know, all
this time they held her tightly, whether or not it was safe to
laugh, or possibly just to smile.

Hallelujah, they called out and bundled her into her car and
set out down the turnpike, with one of the young men driving
her car, the other young man following behind in his car, and
both young men talking to one another over their walkie-talkies
or CB radios, praising God and saying to their listeners that
this girl cannot remember who she is and this girl cannot
remember her brother's name and oh, praise God, this girl
cannot remember that we are in the state of Delaware. She
directed the young Witness who drove her car—for, though
she knew no names, she did recall the appearance of the roads
and streets, and so she could tell them how to drive to her
nameless brother's house, more or less at least, doubling back
over cloverleafs and overheads, down along the exit lanes and
around the center strips.

They sped down along the turnpike, then, careering from

lane to lane—for the driver of her car was only sixteen and did not know much about steering or braking—and her new friends sang out the praises of God, shouting in joy, calling out to motorists, Hallelujah and Praise the Lord and God Save Us, amazed in the presence of the inexplicable, awestruck by the power of the unknown, joyful in the care of the Lord, praying and declaiming into their CB radios. And that, she said, was when I knew I was losing my mind.

Two

She was fine for several months afterward and finally dismissed her episode with the Jehovah's Witnesses as a passing curiosity until, in February, back at the Manhattan School of Music—where she always noticed, as everyone there always noticed, watching carefully, aware and self-aware, self-absorbed, observant, the way fellow performers would speak and move, the way that they would stand and sing, breathe, expand the diaphragm, purse the lips, set the embrasure, elevate the chin, place the foot just so, hold the hands at recital—her brain abruptly shook her and threw her to the floor. At first her right hand trembled and then her arm; her right leg shivered and convulsed, as she watched, puzzled at first, and then terrified. Her side fluttered, her stomach, her flanks, buttocks; her arm thrashed; her head was thrown furiously against her shoulder, flailing, crashing against herself.

So, her mother used to say when she was a child, when she would have a tantrum, crying and kicking, when her mother had despaired, having tried before to hold her, to comfort her, sometimes to cry with her, having declared at last to her father that nothing would calm the child, so, her mother said finally, you're on stage again, are you?

She awoke to find herself surrounded by teachers and friends, ambulance drivers, supporting players, students, the dean, Dean Witford, supernumeraries, and the chorus teacher, the man who copied out the lyrics in his delicate cursive script, hovered there, and she was helped to her feet and walked out, white-coated men on each side, to the ambulance, parked out in front of the main entrance of the school on 122nd Street, a few yards up from Broadway, near The Riverside Church, she, the star, said, as they helped her into the back of the ambulance, as the audience crowded around, I'm fine, thank you. It's okay. Don't worry, I'm fine.

They closed the door behind her, blonde and especially lovely with her cheeks flushed from the seizure and the sudden rush into the winter air. It had been, by far, the most brilliant performance of the academic year, and it might even have been, as the astounded would-be thespians may have thought, really real—though that was not certain.

On the way back down Broadway, past Columbia University, to St. Luke's Hospital, she checked her name, saying to herself quietly over and over, I am Kathy Morris; my name is Kathy Morris. I am Kathy Morris. And she considered her symptoms to see what pattern they divulged: a loss of memory, of sense of self, name, place, and so forth, and a seizure— vague and inconclusive, they were; not definitive, perhaps unrelated, merely random quirks, nothing serious.

I'm really okay, you know, she said to the attendant who rode with her in the ambulance. I'm really perfectly fine. My name is Kathy Morris. The attendant did not seem to be impressed, and so she said, my brother's name is Patrick, my uncle's name is Jeremy, his wife's name is Abigail, my head, you see, is perfectly together.

During the past year Jay had noticed that she had been irritable at times, at times depressed. She had eaten too much. She had gained weight. She had gotten almost fat—not quite, not exactly fat, not terribly fat anyway, but fattish, plump so to say, chubby, perhaps is the right word although that suggests babyishness. Perhaps she had been slightly babyish during the past year too, she thought—regressive in some sense; childish, at least. She had been childish. She could remember one or two instances at least of definite childishness that could still make her face feel hot. She had been pessimistic at times, too. She had once threatened to kill herself, once, when Jay had gone to Atlanta for a time. One should be chary of such threats, for the body is an extraordinary thing that picks up hints and transforms them into such things as cancer, emphysema, broken legs, ulcers, hypertension, heart attacks, strokes perhaps. She had spent too much money during the past year, and she had eaten like a pig. She had been utterly irrational at times—being the very essence of sweetness with Jay one day, bitter and enraged the next day. She had been volatile, out of control at times. She played games a lot, and lied. She had lied quite a lot to Jay when she had begun dating Alvin. She had lied to them both in fact, all the time, every day, ten or twenty times a day. Now this was God's punishment for lying. Of course that was stupid, but such things can never be told absolutely for certain. She was late for all her appointments; she kept messing up whole days at a time, starting out late, getting later, missing dates, standing people up, going home to bed. She felt crazy at times, at times completely crazy. She did not show up for classes some days, sometimes for days in a row; she was failing some courses. She forgot things.

These were her symptoms. It was not clear to her just which ones she positively needed to report to the doctor, or in what order she ought to report them.

Three

She had been to St. Luke's before to visit school friends: the piano player who had smashed up his car on Riverside Drive, the saxophonist who had fallen down during a performance, a drummer knifed and rolled early in the morning outside the jazz club near Columbia. She knew the hospital vaguely, its green and orange visitors' passes, chalk green corridors, wards, private and semiprivate rooms, but she had not been in the emergency room before.

She wished she had entered the hospital through the other door up near Morningside Drive on 113th Street, just across the street from the sanctuary of the grand old pile of the Cathedral of St. John the Divine, the entrance that opened into the old WASP bastion of the hospital with its light-headed high ceilings, windows like those of the Century Club that gave out on a swooning view down across Central Park, back toward the East Side. Here the rich entered, the little old ladies helped out of Lincoln Continentals, Mercedes Benzes, Rolls Royces even, Episcopalians and Presbyterians, escorted by solicitous husbands, sleek and righteous, silver-haired, horn-rimmed, pin-striped, members of the board, clipped and pink, Huntingtons, Burkes, Clarks, Mrs. Fowlkes and Mr. Iselin, Eben Pyne and A. Varick Stout, all of too solid stock and character to fall ill—but all of whom maintained the hospital, just in case—and out of charity. The hospital had been founded—all the plaques agreed, she observed—by the Episcopal minister William Augustus Muhlenberg in 1850 as a church hospital to care for the poor, and although it had acquired a reputation also for the treatment of complications arising from tension, overeating, and sitting too much, the hospital was now stranded at last among the poor and desperate of Harlem, with an ugly modern wing facing Amsterdam Avenue and the Upper West Side, where its emergency entrance received the fractured skulls, head trauma, gunshot wounds, neglect, frostbite, ratbite, filth, malnutrition, rage, bitterness, abrupt hemorrhage of membranes, slash wounds, puncture wounds.

They die, she thought, as she was chaperoned through the door of the emergency entrance, these people die, at early ages, without teeth, snuffling, oozing pus, filthy, crooked, hunched, bent, and twisted, dressed in brown and black, old people, hairless, giving off a stink of decay—blacks and Puerto Ricans most of them, living off welfare, homeless some of them, drunk, hopped-up, red-eyed, slavering, crazy many of them, condemned to sit and wait and die in wards and clinics. She did not wish to be condemned with these pathetic, horrible, loathsome mortal crowds without fathers or mothers to care for them (PACIENTES SOLAMENTE, NO ACOMPAÑANTES), without the proper contacts, people who knew about doctors, white friends, people with money to pay doctors' bills, insure the best possible care, spare no expense, who cares what it costs as long as it saves my daughter; she did not want to be submerged, no, nameless in this hopeless mass of slow death.

The doctor's hands were clean, and his fingernails were neatly trimmed, and he kept her attention distracted from the ruined and the desperate, the stainless steel, the chalk green, odor of disinfectant, cashier's desk, policeman with the handlebar mustache, the open wound, the blood. He asked questions quietly and spoke of epilepsy only to deny its plausibility; she was too old to show the first symptoms now; she had no history of seizures, grand or petit; and so forth. Other doctors came to look at her, to ask a question or two, to stand by, residents and interns, orderlies. She was pretty, and she was hurt, vulnerable, a willing patient, trusting and alone, wishing to be taken care of; she was blonde, and her eyes were blue-green, her voice was soft and rich, full and ebbing, a mezzo-soprano, warm and comforting, encompassing and nestling; it was her voice that drew everyone in and held them—not the doctors alone, but the nurses, too, crowded around her, touched her hand, shoulder, cheek, brushing quickly, lingering only a moment or two, just so. She was young, their age, and she was a charm, or omen, to them.

In time, she was taken back through the battleship gray-green corridors, past microchemistry, biochemistry, bacteriology, electrophoresis, men's room, radiochemistry, assistant pathologist, pathologist, janitor, women's room, stock room, air-conditioning equipment, closet, stairway, records, records, records, preparation, cytology, urinalysis, tissue, tissue culture, and hematology into the Computer Assisted Tomography Scan room, quiet, humidity- and temperature-controlled, soft to the skin, with silent softly colored red and green lights scattered among the banks of computer consoles, and into the adjoining room of white walls, white sound, a wheeled pallet,

spare and covered with a clean white sheet, and the great, fat,
six-foot-high square plastic doughnut—a great powdered
doughnut with a perfectly round hole in its center. It, too, was
white and soundless. She lay down on the pallet, and her head
was held immobile by the stainless steel clamps, lightly
padded, she lightly sedated, and, again, the doctors gathered,
and the interns, and the nurses and orderlies, watching her as
the wheeled pallet was moved slowly into the center of the
doughnut. The scanner worked its way discreetly around her
head, shooting thousands of X-ray beams from diverse angles,
beams that would be resolved by the computer into several
dozen black and white photographic pictures of slices, each
eight millimeters thick, of her head. She felt nothing, heard
nothing. She slept. She had been on stage from the earliest
age, from the time she had been five or six years old. She sang.
Her mother, a pretty woman, would dress her, and she would
sing, for family parties, for school assemblies, for other occasions she had forgotten.

When she was ten years old, and her mother was sick, she
took care of the house after school. She straightened up her
own room, her brother's room, she cooked dinner, she
straightened up the living room and in the morning, she made
breakfast. After a time, she cried. She could not take care of
her whole family, she said. Someone would have to take care
of *her*. Her mother, she said, would have to get a maid. And
the next morning when she awoke, she heard the terrible crash
upstairs and ran up to find her mother on the floor. Her mother
had tried to make the beds but was too weak and had fallen and
now could not get up.

And then she was taken with some sense of purposiveness
(what is it?), some sense of end in view, back along the corridors (men's room, stairway, elevator, women's room) to an

examining room where she sat—how long? an hour?—until
Russ came into the room and sat down with his pencil and
clipboard.

> 82-49-86
> Morris, Kathy
> 306 Riverside Drive, Apartment 8A, New York, New
> York
> Father's name: Patrick
> Mother's name: Catherine Heffron
> Nearest friend or relative: Friend: Alvin Fredericks,
> Apartment 8A, 306 Riverside Drive. Brother Patrick lives at
> 8523 Brae Bridge, Wilmington, Delaware (302-552-2787)
> This is the 1st St. Luke's Hospital admission for this 22-
> year-old white female who presents with onset of seizure
> activity. ROS: Insignificant. PMH: no unusual childhood dis-
> eases. Had tonsil operation, allergic to PCN. Told of a heart
> murmur on school physicals. MDS: Taking erythromycin,
> Tylenol, and codeine (for recent root canal) which, she says,
> "spaced her out." VS—BP 110/70. L arm Supine P 100
> (what is it?). Skin—unremarkable. Neck—supple.
> Carotids—good. Lymphatics no involvement. Breasts—
> small; no masses, nipples everted. Lungs—clear to P & A.
> (what is it?). Abdomen sound, no masses. Pelvic—receives
> regular checkup for IUD. (Shall I put my clothes back on?)
> Patient lives with boyfriend, does own cooking and shop-
> ping, takes no drugs—none?—alcohol only socially, does not
> smoke, has regular sleeping habits, elimination.
> Would really like to get down to about 116 pounds.

She had no secrets left. The lights in the examining room
were bright, and she felt as naked as if her eyelids had been
permanently held open with adhesive tape.

> Patient's mother died ten years ago at age 31, of cancer;
> patient's father died two years ago at age 47 of cardiovascular
> accident; grandfather died six weeks ago of cancer.

Would you like to put this on?

What is it?

It's just a temporary gown.

What?

Patient had elective abortion at age 17.

I don't think of it as a person, you know. Jay just doesn't talk about it at all. It was not a baby to me. It was nothing, you know, I mean, it was not a baby; I'm just not able to deal with the feeling of it being a baby. It was something we went through, something we had to get out.

Objectively the patient has a Class IV lesion on brain scan in the L temporal region in the early uptake phase.

What is it?

Well, we can't say for sure just yet, but I think we can rule out epilepsy. It looks as though there is something in there.

What?

A foreign object of some kind.

Where?

In your head.

She should, perhaps, have said she lived with Jay so that the hospital would notify him of her seizure. Living with Alvin had turned out to be a mistake in any case. It had been almost inadvertent. She wished she lived with Jay, and this address she gave on Riverside Drive was not, in any real sense, her true address but only the result of hurt feelings and confusion, inexperience and a need to be consoled, a misunderstanding and some inability to determine who ought to make a decision in a crisis and who ought to insist or pretend not to care or to leave such questions freely to one another or take charge as a father might—but they had moved along to other questions by this time, and it was too late.

I wish I could get my clothes on.

We'd like to keep you here in the hospital overnight so we can do a few more tests early tomorrow morning.

Why?

You'll need to sign this.

What does it say?

It's just an admission slip.

What is it in my head?

We don't know for sure.

What's your guess?

We don't like to guess. We'll do more tests.

Right. I don't think I can, you know, sign this. I mean, because, you know my hand is shaking.

Right. Take your time.

(A silence.)

I think I'd better just print it, okay?

Right. That's fine.

Four

Admission
Date 2/19 Time 4:00 P.M. Method: Walking
Disposition of valuables: None
Financial class: Self-pay

What is this?

This is your room.

What are these people doing in there?

They share your room.

I wish I had my own room.

Well, no one on the ward service has a private room.

I don't want to go in there.

It's just a room.

I don't think I'll go in.

You have the same doctors, the same nurses, the same X-rays, the same everything. You just share a room.

Those people are dying.

No, they're not.

Look at that woman, will you look at her, hanging upside down? Why is she hanging upside down?

She's in traction.

Why is she upside down?

Well, that's . . .

She's dying. That woman is dying. I'm not going to go in there and spend the rest of my life watching that woman die.

Listen . . .

All of them are dying. All these people are absolutely dying. I am not being stuffed in this ward and die like a nigger.

This is . . .

Is that woman going to die?

Is she . . .

Is she going to die or isn't she?

She . . .

Is that other woman going to die? Look at her! That woman is dying! Oh, God, is she looking at me?

I love you! the woman cried.

What's that?

I love you!

Hey, lady, are you speaking to me?

I love you!

Oh, God . . .

Hey, listen . . .

I'm getting out of here. . . .

Wait up.

Five

She sat quietly for a while, then, downstairs in one of the examination rooms. Cold outside. Darkening midwinter mid-afternoon. She thought she might go to another hospital if there were not another room for her at St. Luke's; she said as much to a passing nurse and later on to a passing doctor and even later, she said the same to the intern Russ when he stood at the door to say hello.

She inspected her hospital gown and hospital bathrobe in detail—their wrinkles, myriad, like old skin, so often washed. She considered the floor and tried to guess whether it had been scrubbed an hour before, or two hours before, whether it had been scrubbed as a matter of routine or because someone had bled on it, whether someone had died in that room that afternoon. Again evening came. She considered the desk, the walls, chalk green, the door.

A kind doctor entered then and sat down, saying nothing but hello. He had her chart, and he read it. It was very quiet.

I want to leave.

Yes.

I don't want to be in that room with those people.

I know.

May I leave?

You could, yes.

But I have something in my head.

Yes.

What is it, a tumor?

Yes.

What are we going to do?

Take it out.

Do you know, I'm just a girl, well, a young woman really, but I'm not accustomed to this. I don't have brain tumors every day, and I don't know how to handle it, you know, I'm doing the best I can, but I don't really want to be in that ward. I don't think I hate blacks much, you know, but I go to school around here, you know, and I see what happens to them, and I don't want to be treated like a piece of garbage; I don't want to be put in the exact same situation as those dying niggers upstairs—am I getting through to you?—I want to be treated as a person, you know, because I absolutely do not have any intention at all in any way whatsoever or in any other form of doing absolutely anything at all but staying completely and completely alive, absolutely and terrifically alive, you know what I mean? Nobody's killing me.

Right. Maybe we can get another room tomorrow. Meantime, you can stay in the ward.

(A long silence.)

Right. Thanks. Listen, you tell everyone what I said, okay? All the nurses and the other doctors and everyone, will you? Do I have your attention? What I said about staying alive, okay?

Right.

Six

He thought he might be taken for a secret agent by the toll booth operator at the George Washington Bridge. He wondered whether a stranger would consider him an ordinary person as he came into Manhattan early each morning, so early that the sun had not risen—and his features were, he knew, obscured somewhat by the steam of his breath, and rendered entirely indecipherable by the shadow cast by the greenish neon lights at the toll booth—or whether he would be perceived somehow as a man who was, by profession, always just next to the possibility of something dangerous.

He, Cunnought, had known operatives—of a sort, anyhow: his uncle who was always traveling in Eastern Europe and who everyone said might just be an agent; a professional acquaintance who had conducted drug experiments in an Upper West Side brownstone some years ago; and, best of all, an old college roommate who had made a specialty of concocting poisons out of snake venom and rare herbs for the Company, a fellow known now as Mr. Death.

He regarded the clues. He drove a maroon Datsun with a broken seat belt and a broken driver's seat that needed to be propped up and held in place by boxes. (He could make nothing of that.) He drove fast, cutting off other drivers, happily in and out of lanes—a cowboy, a Genghis Khan of the highways, one of the last of the individualists, utterly alone in this adventure of crossing the great Hudson, as in an antique engraving.

An acquaintance of his had climbed Everest only a few months before. Two men were chosen for the final assault on the peak, the two best climbers. At the top, the temperature drops far below zero, and the winds are fierce, and the two men became intoxicated as they approached the peak. In order to return safely to their base camp before dark, before they would be hopelessly lost in the wind and cold of the night, they had to reach the peak by three fifteen in the afternoon and then start back down almost at once. If they were not on their proper schedule, they would be obliged to turn back. By three fifteen, they were not yet near the top. Members of the climbing party back down along the mountain watched through binoculars as their two best men continued upward. At four fifteen the two climbers were spotted on the peak, marking their triumph with a flag placed firmly in the snow. After dark, the temperature fell to fifty degrees below zero, Fahrenheit, and the winds reached sixty miles per hour. At dawn, no search party needed to be sent up Everest to find the bodies. The two climbers were spotted emerging well-rested from their tent: they had returned to their camp in the dark; they had memorized their way along the ridges of snow and ice.

He needed a haircut, like all cowboys. Like all cowboys, he had no time for such petty stuff, and he rarely combed his hair either. And yet he observed other conventions punctiliously.

He was clean-shaven. He wore a light gray herringbone tweed sport coat, a shirt with light blue stripes, a dark red tie sporting mallards in flight, dark charcoal gray slacks, brown loafers. What else? He was forty years old. He tended toward stockiness, with a face that appeared babyish at times, and at other times like the face of the prizefighting son of a Welsh coal miner, a face with lumps of muscle, a gum chewer's face, a face that betrayed glimpses of incipient distinction, which would, in old age, look ravaged and, beneath a flourish of white hair, distinguished. His eyes darted from side to side, habitually alert, excited, and relishing whatever they saw, whether the colors of the rising sun or the surface of the road ahead, the light reflected from the snow and ice and the windowpanes of Harlem, the storefronts, tenement stoops, or the ironwork of the elevated train as it emerges from under the ground at 125th Street.

When he had been a resident at the Neurological Institute, he had operated to remove a low-grade malignant tumor from the cranium of a twelve-year-old girl. Before the operation her vision had been failing and afterward, as she awaited radiotherapy, her vision continued to deteriorate. She knew something was going wrong with her eyes, but she did not want to go back into the operating room; and so, in order to pass the eye examinations that the doctors gave her, she memorized the eye chart. Puzzled by the erratic symptoms she displayed, he tapped into her spine and drained some of the cerebrospinal fluid. Within four hours the young girl had gone absolutely blind.

He parked in the doctors' parking lot in the shadow of the Cathedral of St. John the Divine, across the street from the Main Entrance to St. Luke's Hospital, the entrance he always used. A sedate, fringed canopy covers the short walkway here to the several steps and the grand double doors, a half-dozen marble steps and then the central hall that is surmounted by a miniature rotunda. Directly ahead is the hospital's chapel, with stained glass windows of Christ the Consoler and the Seven Acts of Mercy.

In Texas, his brother told him, you can hire a hit man for five hundred dollars. But, someone had said, I wouldn't kill anyone for five thousand dollars. What is the difference between a physician and a sociopath? A psychiatrist, Cunnought said, must take chances. A psychiatrist who has never had a patient commit suicide is not a good psychiatrist; he is keeping his patients too safely under lock and chain and not letting them grow. A good surgeon has complications. A good surgeon, so the joke goes, can make a living taking care of his complications. If a surgeon produces no complications, he is too conservative; he is not operating at the limits of knowledge and skill; he is not fierce enough to risk finding the answer somewhere in the unknown; he is too frightened of wiping out, too timid to stay out there for long, tracing the edge of chaos, risking falling over the edge into catastrophe, confusion, disorder, terror, and death, like the slalom champion who triumphs by a hundredth of a second because he dares to press to the very edge of possibility, skittering along, defining the very line that runs along both order and disorder, life and death. The difference is that a sociopath relishes death.

The doctors' lounge is reassuring, comforting to Cunnought like a small dining hall at Yale, or something smaller, a senior common room. One needs a key to enter the pale doors of this room, with the fireplace at the far end, small desks along the walls, a large table in the center, white walls, eggshell white with delicate carved cornices around its lofty ceiling, and portraits of great physicians, now dead, placed firmly at intervals.

In 1915, Cunnought's grandfather had performed an autopsy on a thirteen-year-old girl and discovered the cause of
diabetes—an act that nearly won for him the Nobel Prize.
Harvey Cushing had chosen Grandpapa to go on the yellow
fever expedition during the Spanish-American War. Later on,
he had been one of the original scientists at The Rockefeller
University. He told stories of having lunch with John, and of the
times that Nelson had to wait on the table. He lived to the age
of ninety-seven. Toward the end, he was very hard of hearing
and almost blind. He had to be led to his office each day; even
so, even then, he continued to turn out papers for the medical
journals. Cunnought was finishing his residency then. Grandpapa invited him to dinner one night and asked him how old he
would be when he finished his residency. Thirty-five, Cunnought answered proudly, having attended Haverford, Yale,
the University of Pennsylvania medical school, studied psy-
chiatry, served as a psychiatrist in the Army, switched to neurosurgery and thus arrived at the moment he was ready to put
all his training into practice. What had Grandpapa been doing
at the age of thirty-five? Grandpapa answered in confusion and
embarrassment: at the age of thirty-five, he was already dean
of the medical school at Washington University in St. Louis.

White-coated, Cunnought walked the marble corridor to the
meeting room where the weekly Friday neurological conference was held, where the house staff presented interesting
cases, patients whose difficulties did not easily yield to diagnosis, old wrecks whose neurological deficits had become so
obscured by psychological problems, compensatory strategies,
coverups, and other evasions as to have become enshrouded in
mystery. Somewhere, underlying the stumbling gait, the uncertain vision, the ignorance of time and place, of the name of
the hospital or of the current President of the United States, the

speech that rambled on in perfect cadence, marked by impeccable syntax but entirely devoid of meaning, somewhere lay the irreducible facts of neuronal connections, synapses, chemical and electrical interactions, the quick passage of sodium ions—although the presence even of these seeming realities was obscure and perhaps, finally, merely provisional or fantastical.

Cunnought's father just lives and breathes medicine, Cunnought says; he leaves the house every morning at seven fifteen and comes home about eight o'clock at night. He has a very large practice. He's a psychiatrist in Philadelphia. He started out as a physiologist, graduated from medical school, and actually went into physiology and did a lot of experiments in neurophysiology. I went to medical school with the idea of being a psychiatrist. I felt a strong identification with him. He has tremendous energy and terrific high spirits, very quick, and very direct.

He was one of Grandpapa's research students, and that was when he met my mother. He married the boss's daughter. I grew up in a family of eight children. My family have little time for anything except medicine. One brother is an orthopedist, one a gastroenterologist, and one has just finished his medical residency at Cornell.

In fact, originally there were nine children; one was born with a neurological deficit—an exposed spinal cord, not even covered by skin. Fortunately my parents were very sophisticated people; they just didn't try to do a thing to save the child; they just let it go.

When we were children, we always played sports. There was tremendous competitiveness.

My mother would always sit in the background keeping people happy.

My mother is a serenely quiet woman. She never gets angry.
She was always a peacemaker.

We used to have, the children in my family, tremendous
fights. It wasn't unusual for us to throw stones at each other,
hitting each other in the head. One day the phone rang, and
one of my brothers answered and said he couldn't get my
mother because she had locked herself in the bedroom.

My parents always had one or two maids.

It was an elegant life.

My mother drove us to school, to Haverford, every morning. Once there were six of us in Haverford at the same time.
Imagine the incredible expense of that for my father. I didn't
appreciate it at the time. We all played football and soccer and
baseball, and my mother used to drive us to school in the
morning, and to the games, and we would all get together for
Sunday dinners with the family, and it was chaos. Chaos.
Wonderful.

Other than that we'd see Dad when he came home at night.

When Janet and I were married, my mother took her aside
several times and asked her whether she realized what she was
getting into. But Janet was an avid reader. I'm not at all, but
she is. She went to Smith, and she loves to read, I don't know
how many books in a week. She's always been that way. She's
always been able to spend a great deal of time by herself, and
she enjoys it. She's not very social. I mean, if we don't have to
go to a party, it doesn't upset her at all. Frequently, during my
residency, I used to get home at nine or ten o'clock at night,
and we'd go to a party, and I'd just fall asleep.

(He could not be sure whether she was sure he loved her.)

Correll, one of the neurosurgeons from the Neurological
Institute, once fell asleep while he was flying his own small
plane. His wife, who was with him on the trip, looked up from

her book and noticed he had put the plane on automatic pilot so
that he could take a quick nap. She never flew with him again.
Correll loved more than anything to be in the operating room.
He just loved it. He loved it the way I do. When I was doing
my residency at the Neurological Institute, someone said to
me, Get ready, Correll's coming back, and I asked what he
meant, and he said that Correll was returning from vacation
that night, and he would be wanting to get into the operating
room. He had patients all over the place, and, whenever
anyone else canceled out of an operation, he would take the
booking for the operating room and move one of his patients
in. I remember finishing an operation with him one time, for a
meningioma, at about eleven o'clock at night, and he asked me
to close because he wanted to go downstairs and look at a
patient. I just knew he would be bringing that patient up to the
operating room. He just hadn't had enough for that particular
night.

I get home at nine or ten o'clock still quite a lot. I didn't
realize how often I worked so late until one night I got home in
time for dinner. We used to eat dinner in a breakfast room, and
it was a little crowded, so Janet had pushed the table back
against the wall to make more room. I got home one night for
dinner, and then we realized: the place that had been pushed
against the wall—that was my place. I hadn't been home for
dinner for two months.

He was told at the neurological conference that a young
woman with a possible brain tumor would have an angiogram
done that morning. To have heard of a gunshot wound would
have depressed him, a definitely malignant tumor would have
been bad; but to hear simply of a tumor, one that might not be
malignant, offered the wonderful prospect of some fine hours
in the operating room, of some fun, some excitement, some

interest, and of the chance of a cure. Cunnought thought, as a colleague at the Neurological Institute used to say: that's great, old man, great, that's just great. Two neurosurgeons were on the medical staff at St. Luke's, and they took on whatever cases stumbled into the hospital requiring surgery—as well as bringing their own private patients to the hospital. On this morning, Cunnought was the neurosurgeon present, and so he took the case.

Seven

The sheet of film on which the angiogram is developed is heavy and thick and comes out of the developing solution a rich black, except for the delicate white shadow of the skull, so surprisingly small, and manifestly fragile, transparent in some places and translucent in others, crisply limned in yet other places as though it had suddenly condensed into stratus clouds, or, elsewhere, into the hard edge of porcelain; and, within that inconstant outline, deep within the blackness, are the crisp white arcs of the arteries that have been filled, for the few seconds needed to memorialize this vision, with a radioactive substance. The massive carotid artery rises from the heart and branches suddenly into myriad smaller vessels, and those branch in turn into fine tendrils, and those, finally, in their turn, into the finest of traceries that arch and pulse and leap in extraordinarily intricate and surprising patterns, as though they danced through the brain.

Although at first these lines seem random, impulsive, improvisational, each one has a particular goal and pathway, and

it is by noticing how a given artery deviates from its path—
how this artery vaults too high or that artery curves too tightly
and gracelessly—that one can deduce the presence of a foreign
body in the skull.

In the case of Kathy Morris, in a place in her left temporal
lobe, just behind her temple, just above and in front of her left
ear, the angiogram shows an embarrassed blush. No blood
vessels, great or small, leap through this space; no bright arcs of
blood dance here. Instead there is confusion; there is a chaos of
blood vessels that is disquieting, and that is not beautiful.

The blush is the mark of a tumor, a small, gnarled fist of
tissues—unmistakable in its alien ugliness, an ugliness unlike
anything else, whether bloody or viscous, inside the body—
and the sight, even of its indistinct shadow on the angiogram, is
appalling. It does not nurture the brain, nor protect it. It does
not bring the rich nourishment of blood to it nor help to bathe it
with the cerebrospinal fluid. It does not contribute to the functioning of the brain; nor does it appear itself to cogitate. It only
kills. It kills more or less slowly and with absolute certainty—unless it is killed first. Whether it took up this space
a year before or twenty years before is unknown. How quickly
it has grown to usurp so much space is unknown. Its origins
are unknown.

This tumor, appalling as it may be, is still not the worst of
all possible tumors. The shadow it casts on the angiogram is
encouraging: no major blood vessels run through it, and so, in
removing the tumor, it will not be necessary to risk destroying
any large vessels, which would destroy the blood supply to a
part of the brain and perhaps destroy that part of the brain. The
tumor, large as it may be, is compact; the angiogram does not
show traces of tumor elsewhere in the brain: this tumor seems

to be nonmalignant. And it is on the surface of the brain, not deep within the brain, but just adhering to the surface of the left temporal lobe: it is a meningioma; and, if one is to have a tumor at all, this is the best of all possible tumors to have. It is, compared to the others, a lark of a tumor.

Not long before, Cunnought had operated on an eighty-six-year-old woman who had a meningioma near the midline, where it might have been tangled up with vessels leading to the brain stem. While he was taking it, Cunnought said, he got into a lot of bleeding and so he had to bring it out quickly so that he could stuff cotton down into the hole and try to stop the bleeding. The worst thing in any operation is uncontrolled bleeding. Janet saw a cardiac surgeon on television one time when he was asked what he feared most in the operating room, and he said without a moment's hesitation, uncontrolled bleeding. That is what any surgeon fears. Control the bleeding. That's first. I must control the bleeding. I stop it first just by throwing in cotton and then, once I've stopped it, I come back very slowly and peel away the cotton very gently and cauterize any vessels I see bleeding, taking care not to sacrifice a vessel that will kill a patient. Control the bleeding: that's first; control the bleeding, or you've lost your grasp on the patient's life; it slips away, then; you've lost control, you've stumbled into death.

But I just went ahead to get the tumor out quickly so that I could get down into the bleeding, and it just turned out to be duck soup; all of a sudden it just came out. All of a sudden it just rolled out; it rolled out onto the table, and I just looked at it, and as I looked at it, it just rolled off the table and right onto the floor. Somebody said what's that, and I said it's a tumor, and they just stood around and looked at it. A lot of people in the room had never seen a brain tumor, and they looked at it, and they all stood back from it for a long time. No one wanted to touch it.

And I went down and stopped the bleeding; it turned out to be a snap, and an operation that should have taken six hours only took two hours. And the lady did very well. She woke up right after the operation and I said How are you, and she said, Fine thanks, and how are you? I was great. I felt just great. Just great, I said. I told her, I'm just great.

But this operation on Kathy Morris was going to be even better. Cunnought noticed that a lot of extra people were standing around and looking at the film. He had heard that the patient was a young woman, and he had passed a good-looking young woman in the waiting room outside, and then he thought yes, there were four or five extra people standing around looking at the angiogram, and he knew absolutely yes she is going to enjoy her time in the hospital, everyone is going to enjoy her being in the hospital, everyone is going to get involved with her case, and she is going to get a lot of attention and a lot of care, and she doesn't quite know that she is seducing them, and they are telling themselves that they are learning about an interesting medical case, but they are all young, she is, and the interns and residents are, and the nurses are, and they are all going to have a wonderful time together. Once a girl was brought into the Neurological Institute. A beautiful girl. He had never seen more medical students interested in a diagnosis. Working her up. Sitting down tapping her reflexes. It was great. And, when she was presented at rounds, somebody asked her what she wanted to be when she finished school, and she said Well, she was very interested in helping people, and she wanted to do something in sex education.

Now, looking at Kathy Morris' X-ray, they shook their heads

saying, oh that's terrible and oh my God, and he asked them to
tell him about her. They told him that she had presented with a
background of a couple of seizures and how old she was and
that sort of thing, and then they said, and she's a senior at the
Manhattan School of Music, and she is about to graduate and,
from what they hear, she is supposed to be really a very good
singer, and then he thought Oh my God, because the tumor
was in the left temporal lobe, and that is where the speech
center is located, and, even though a meningioma is duck
soup, there is always the chance that he would have to take a
blood vessel, perhaps, in peeling the tumor off the surface of
the brain, and that might infarct the speech area, and they said
to him, well, what are you going to do, and will she be okay,
and he was not ready to answer questions like that just at the
moment, and it sort of teed him off, so he said, Well, I'll just
take it out and maybe she'll die, and maybe she'll never speak
again, or maybe I won't have to remove more than ''Smoke
Gets in My Eyes,'' and then he turned around and walked out
to the waiting room where she was.

The young interns who had never encountered Cunnought
before were shocked by him. They were accustomed to being
taught their medicine by older, tranquil doctors who had long
since learned to overcome or hide their feelings, and Cunnought's quick passions took them by surprise. His en-
thusiasms and his disappointments, and the black humor he
used to cover up his anger, were all matters of intense curiosity. When he was idle, he prowled the corridors to look for
patients to take into the operating room; when operations went
well he bragged and when they went badly he let everyone
know just exactly what went wrong, and when there was nothing that he could do when he saw someone dying, he turned
bitter, mocking, and ironic. If he were phoned in the middle of

the night—merely as a matter of routine—to be asked about a
case, a gunshot wound, or a man who had fallen from the top
of a building, when everyone knew that it was hopeless, that
the patient was sure to die and the only question was one of
time, Cunnought would tell the resident on duty: just put him
in the control group.

On his desk, in his office, he had a plastic model of
three vertebrae. He treated it without reverence; he used it
as a pencil holder. And still, he did not wish to lose himself behind a façade of black humor. He labored hard to
stay in touch with his unrestrained feelings. Too many
doctors spent their lives anesthetized against the pain of
their daily lives. Cunnought had to get himself up to enter
the operating room. It was a place he loved more than any
other and yet, people died too often there. One had to
avoid battle fatigue. So often he stood at the head of the
table and watched someone die—someone of his mother's
age, his father's age, someone of Janet's age. He told a
resident once, who stood beside him in the operating room,
asking just how the surgeon thought he could best define
the concept of death: You will know what dead means
when you've killed someone.

I thought she was very attractive, he said later. I'm not part
of the flirtatious young gang of interns any more, but—what
the hell—I thought it was too bad. She was young to have a
tumor.

I went over to her then, where she was lying on a cart, and I
was about to speak to her when one of the nurses stepped
between us and said to her, This is your neurosurgeon, Dr.
Cunnought. And I was about to say something then when she
said, Well, at least you're handsome. I wanted to be very
serious; it would have been fun to flirt then, to say something

amusing, but eventually, she and I knew, I would be inside her
head, and she did not want me to be light-hearted then, and so
I asked her very quietly, how was your angiogram? Did it hurt
you? And she was quiet then and very direct, and she said no,
it was not bad.

She thought that he was very young and very good-looking.
She was comforted to know that he was a Celt as she was, but
she had wished he would be older and not handsome at all. All
at once I could imagine him playing tennis, and I wished I
could not see him on the tennis court. Of course, he was good
on the court, but only an average player, really. He could not
be best at everything—and what he was best at was surgery. I
wished he were older and that he didn't play tennis and that all
he did was practice surgery, but I suppose he needed to relax
now and then, to rest so that he would be ready to operate. I
thanked him for asking about the angiogram, and I asked him
how he ever got into surgery, and he answered me, telling me
about the hospitals at which he had been a resident or an
intern, but I didn't listen. This is the guy who's going to cut
me up, I thought, and I thought yes, he can do it, because he's
very good. If he had a wife—I hoped she were a writer or a
dancer, someone strong, because I knew that he was a doctor
first and only secondly a husband, and I hoped he was married
to someone who understood that—as I understood it, because
he and I, he and I are so much alike.

He did not want to discuss her surgery just then in the hall.
She had already been told by one of the young doctors or
nurses that her tumor was a meningioma, and that was enough
for her to absorb at the moment. He said that he would see her
later, and he went back down the hall in search of a telephone
to call the operating room to schedule an operation.

It occurred to her that he used all this—not just the formality of his manner but the informality, too, the good cheer and high spirits, briskness and quick energy, and even his very directness—to stay aloof and cool, untouched and uncommitted: the operative who moves easily through the scene and then is gone before anyone quite knows who he was, the mystery man who seems buoyantly open and turns out to be invisible to his patients—and perhaps, she thought, to his family as well, the man with whom a woman lives a lifetime, without ever touching him deeply, knowing him intimately, hurting him terribly, or scaring him at all.

Eight

Patrick thought he frightened the nurses with his mad eyes and his reddish-brown hair, his vast hulking size, his powerful biceps, triceps, deltoids, the pectorals and serratus magnus, and the gnarled rectus abdominis whose rippling, knotting, flexing bundles showed through the beautiful, smooth obliquus externus abdominis—as could be seen occasionally in the wrestling magazines—and so he tried to put them at ease now that he was a full-fledged adult having reached his twenty-first birthday and so become mature, with his casual, shuffling manner as he came down the hall on Saturday morning, inquiring cheerily, where's my sister, and hi, you know where my sister is, and hi, hey, where is my sister, you know? And, when he rounded the corner at her door, he stopped and leaned against the door jamb of his sister's new and semi-private room (in which she had been installed comfortably alone).

Hey, Kathy, how are you?

Oh, hi, Patty, I'm fine.

Then what are you doing here?

Oh . . .

He thought she was taking the whole matter much too calmly; she was neither panicky nor really calm; she was evasive. She was treating him like her younger brother, saving him from the bad news. Patrick understood that she was playing a part in some play, but he could not offhand guess just what part in which play.

What is this oh hi Patty I'm fine when I just drove all the way up here from Delaware because my sister is dying, and I risk my life driving up here in my old bullshit carwreck and you say oh hi Patty I'm fine.

Oh . . .

What is going on?

Oh, Patty.

I'm scared out of my freaking mind, and I come in and you say, oh, hi, hi, everything is cool, hi, cool, good to see you, well, I'll be going along then, you know, so long, okay, cool—and he sat on his sister's bed.

Oh, Patty, I am fine, you know, it's okay.

Well, I'm glad you're fine, because I'm really scared.

Hey, it's okay, I have a tumor. . . .

I know, see, I talked to Jeremy, and he said, Hey, Patrick, your sister has a tumor, why don't you come over for dinner—and I thought, come over to dinner, who is this? Is my sister dying of cancer? Hey, how about coming over to dinner, we'll have a steak, you know, and baked potatoes, have a glass of wine and talk about Thomas Aquinas, you know.

I'm not dying of cancer, Patty.

Oh, yeah?

I have a tumor, that's all, and it's going to be removed. It is a benign tumor, a tumor called a meningioma, and it will be taken out, and the doctors say it is a very routine operation.

Oh, yeah?

Yeah.

Oh, well, that's good then, huh?

Yeah.

That's really great.

It's okay.

Shit, that's great.

Yeah, it's okay.

Shit.

(A silence.)

You wouldn't lie to me?

Well, Patty, I've seen the doctors, and they told me I had a tumor, and then I had some tests that confirmed it.

What tests?

Like an angiogram.

What's that?

They take you down to the X-ray department on a what-chamacallit on wheels, what do you call it?

A stretcher.

Yeah. They wheel you into this room that has gigantic machines on the walls and on the ceiling, great fat machines, black and shiny, with a lot of stainless steel, all polished like mirrors and very cold, and they strip you down and lay you out on this polished slab, getting ready to zap you and they adjust the table to the right place then and fix your head in steel clamps so it won't move and then they bring in a lot of X-ray plates, locked shut in steel frames, and put them in boxes, and they turn out all the lights first, and focus the X-ray cameras on your head, marking your temples left and right with small orange crosses, here and here, and then the middle of your forehead, so, another cross, and aim their cameras at these crosses. But they want a

picture not of your bones but of your veins, of the arteries and
veins inside your head, and so they must fill all these with some
radioactive dope that shows up on the plate, and this, the
radioactive dope they inject—this is the hard part, this is the part
that hurts—they inject it in the artery in your thigh. But no, not
even that. They open up a small incision on your leg and then
they put a catheter in your leg and feed that catheter up your leg,
way up your artery, all the way up into your heart, inside your
heart—and then out again!—out up the artery in your neck up
toward your brain, and stop, just there, in your neck, having
watched it all the time on a small, closed-circuit television
screen that flashes on from moment to moment the little instant
X-rays that show the catheter making its way up your leg and
into your heart and neck. . . .

Oh, shit . . .

And then, when everything is ready, they put the dye into
this catheter, and shoot it up directly to your head, and then the
X-ray machine goes zap! zap! zap! zap! zap! zap! zap! zap!
zap! and your head burns, it burns from the inside out, like
small furnace fires, chemical fires burning up your brain, like a
head full of kerosene or gasoline, and you think the smoke will
come out your nose and ears and your forehead split just where
they drew the little cross, and then it fades, it eases then, and
fades and then you're lying there, that's all, on the cold slab
again, and the doctor is smiling like a zombie behind his little
lead jacket and saying it's a very good angiogram, a very good
angiogram, that's all it was.

Weren't you scared?

No, not me.

Yeah, wow.

He was a sweet boy, big, with a gift of gab and an embarrassed smile, who spent much time alone, watching televi-

sion, cops and robbers, war movies, science fiction, football games, and reading wrestling magazines, following the fights, practicing his judo from time to time, karate and jiujitsu, all the martial arts including kung-fu and wu-su and tai-chi-chuan, and occasionally, in front of the television set or mirror, he would drop into the stylish postures of ground dragon, monkey, springing leg, yellow mountain, or moving shadow. He knew a move or two from tae kwon do and from aikido and was able to do esoteric breathing exercises and read Dashiell Hammett at the same time. In college, when he attended it, he studied criminology. He drank beer often enough and often enough got drunk, but he never smoked pot or played with any hard drugs and he avoided all bennies and dexies, all speed, especially, because he felt that his mind and thoughts moved too rapidly for him much of the time in any case.

I talked to Jeremy and Abigail, and they're coming.

Right.

They're fine. We talked a lot.

Right.

I had dinner with Jeremy and Abigail.

Right.

Right. Jeremy thinks you're dying.

Right.

He thinks all tumors are cancer.

Well, he's wrong.

Yeah, let's hope so.

He's wrong.

Yeah. So you're not dying.

Right.

Yeah.

Right.

Right. So that's good then. That's just great. It sure scares
me, though, because I don't think I can make it alone.

Then Patrick heard his sister's friend Eileen enter talking of
the New York *Post* and of the friend of a friend who worked
for the New York *Post* and would make certain to plant a story
about how this hospital was staffed by shmucks and sonsof-
bitches for putting Kathy in a ward—what was this now? a
private room? that's great, but nonetheless—for putting her
(originally) in a ward full of terminal cases, cancer, gunshot
wounds, stabbing victims, and the other drek and horrorshow
stuff they write off in hospitals like this place where the
doctors and nurses don't care who dies but—if she had a
father, yes, or someone else to come in here and kick the walls
and shove some people around and take charge, no one would
stuff her into a ward like that, or if she had money, if she had
insurance, or money, or if she were rich, or if she were a
Rockefeller, you know, there would be doctors and nurses all
over the place, and she would get the best I mean the best care
there is.

Then Mary came and brought with her a lot of TV fan
magazines for Kathy to have in the hospital, and the nurse
named Mary Anne came by with the thermometer and Beth,
who had gone to Boston, who was good-looking, Patrick
thought, skinny, with long dark-blonde hair and an oddly
shaped birthmark on her right forearm, a birthmark that went
right around her forearm as far as Patrick could see, although
he could not tell for certain, hard as he tried to get a better
perspective on it, whether the birthmark completely encircled
Beth's arm, and she brought a teddy bear, and then others
came, students from Kathy's school, strangers to Patrick, one
bearing magazines, and another bringing some book about

God and then—Wow!—a book about death and dying, and
then a Judy Collins record.

Patrick grabbed the book about death and dying and held it
behind his back and retreated toward the door, searching for
some final resting place for the offensive tome. I, he said, you
know, have to . . . uh . . . I'll be back in a minute, and he
disappeared and set out down the corridor in desperate quest of
an open window, laundry chute, or elevator shaft. Should he
give it to someone else, just pop into any room, and lay the
book on some other defenseless man or woman and stand there
waiting for the obligatory expressions of gratitude? He might
present it to a nurse, using it as an occasion to ingratiate
himself and invite her out for a drink. Or he might take it
downstairs and leave it casually on a chair in the emergency
room. He could give it to a doctor, saying here, take this killer.
He could use it to bop someone on the head, hit him on the
back of the neck, across the Adam's apple, knock him to the
floor, and hold him down and choke him, break his nose,
smash his eyes.

We had the feeling (Patrick felt) that our father didn't give a
shit for us. He spent his money. He left us unprepared. He was
not a rich man; he was an office worker, selling stuff, and he
spent all he had and left us nothing when he died, no life
insurance, or college money, or any other things, except our
house, a little house, with a mortgage still to pay. He started
dying when our mother started dying, only it took him longer,
that's all, it took him fifteen years. I'd run downstairs to meet
him when he came home from work, and somehow he made
me feel like dirt. If I didn't feel terrible, he'd start shouting,
and he would tear my room apart, throwing things, and then
he'd hit me, he would hit me, he would just hit me.

My grandfather was the powerful one—the immigrant,
standing on the hillside in front of the steel mill, lunchbox in
his hand, two friends at his sides. He was taller, and broader
than his friends; he had black hair, a fierce, huge man who
loved to hug his grandchildren, pick them up, whirl them
around. He survived cobalt treatments, the amputation of a
leg, more radiation, more cutting up, complications of every
sort, drugs and radiation, powerful and angry and booming.

Patrick took the book with him into the men's room and
considered the several places in which he might dispose of the
thing, not neglecting to size up the wastebasket, but holding
back, wishing for some more symbolic place.

Kathy was like my mother to me when I was small. My
mother was a pal to me, and then I needed Kathy, and she took
care of me. We fought, she and I, we fought terribly, and I
loved her so much.

He would argue, my father, and he would take things out on
Kathy, and when Kathy wanted to go to a dance, he'd make
her feel rotten before she left, and I'd get hit, and I would cry
and go to my room, and Kathy would fight with him, and then
she would leave and I'd be all alone.

She'd be out at rehearsals for the school plays every night
she could, that was her way out. She was safe. I had no place
to go, but she went into every school play, every one, and
then, when she graduated from high school, she went straight
off to the music school, she didn't miss a step, that's how she
handled it.

Then I was alone with my father, I couldn't think of any
way out; and I would run downstairs to meet him.

And when I think about him now, I still shake.

He came back down the corridor with the book still in his
hand, thinking of the possibilities for dropping his bomb in the

nurses' station, the cleaning closet, television room, the laundry chute or window once again. He returned to Kathy's room
with the book still in his hand and went directly to her bed and
said, oh yeah, here, Kathy, it's a book I forgot to give to you.

Who brought me this?

I forgot.

Oh.

His father did not drink until his mother died; she had been
pretty, delicate and fair, fragile in a summer dress, robust in
wool, strong-willed and resilient until her spirit was entirely
broken by the cancer and she could only conclude that God had
not been fair to her—and then his father set about to commit
suicide, as quickly as his religion would allow.

Nine

The visitors, Patrick noticed, were all still saying, who will take charge, and how it wasn't fair, and going out to phone their friends and coming back and saying that it isn't fair, and if she had a father none of this would happen, and going out again to phone and drive somewhere, pick someone up, and call the papers, call the doctor, call the priest or call the nurse or call the school and check out this and check out that, school insurance and Medicaid, and saying who will pay? who will pay? If only there were money and mothers and fathers, everything would be okay.

And this girl, Patrick noticed, this skinny black girl came in from somewhere and sat down on Kathy's bed and began to tell her how to get on welfare and how to get on Medicaid, how she'd been on it all her life, and how you get extra money, get on twice, have double the coverage, and all the ins and outs, this girl's in a private room, and she is really beautiful and quick and smart, but her mind is so complicated and devious, and everything she says is so complex that no one else can follow a single word she's saying.

And now the room was full of freaks and dope addicts, Patrick thought, these guys from Kathy's school, and girls, these singers, actors, guys with freaky braids, you know, and smoking joints and popping pills or shooting stuff, I don't know, and going on, you know, rapping all about this and that, and how this guy plays sax, and how this guy got busted, and how this guy paid off this guy and slept with someone and got this gig, you know, at some nightclub. And they're all saying the brain is this, you know, the brain is that, the brain is this and that. They're waiting in line, you know, there's this line of freaks and peeping toms like the third act of some play, you know, passing out, or swooning, and she's saying, you know, it's all okay and not to worry, and everything will be all right, and how she has this tumor and how it's called a meningioma and that's okay, that's the tops, and how they just go ahead and pop it out and all that's cool, and she tells this tale again and over again 45,000 times, and all these people are standing around, you know, shifting from foot to foot and saying, yeah, yeah, oh yeah, wow, this is really real, man, I mean this is really real, but this is real, and poor Kathy, you know, and that I can't handle, that poor Kathy and this is really real, and she is giving a performance I've never seen before, and she was beautiful, and I could see why they all came to see her and touch her and crowd around her because she was so fierce and so strong and so sweet, and I was scared absolutely petrified.

Then Alvin came, and I hated him, the sneaky little fucker, and I wished he wasn't there. It didn't seem right to me somehow. He treated her almost as if he were her husband, you know, and that seemed wrong to me, and I couldn't even get

close to her. It's not that I hated for her to have a boyfriend. I
like Jay, and I wished he were there instead of Alvin, and
Alvin just stood there, you know, looking cool and sort of
nodding, standing there and sort of nodding, like everything is
cool and everything will be okay. He has this mustache, you
know, and this hairdo that looks like Prince Valiant, and
stands there going, cool, you know, cool, and he says to her
you know, you're a tough lady, and you're going to make it,
you've got to fight, and she says, I know. I am. You're right.
And I wanted to punch his face in.

And then Jay came, and he came in and he sat down on her
bed, and he just cried, you know, that's all he did. I guess he
held her hand and, you know, held her a little bit, and he just
cried, and neither one of them said a word, they didn't have to
talk, and I thought, you know I wish she'd tell him that she
needs him and that she wants him, because I know that's what
she's thinking, that she wants him to stay with her. I don't
know why they ever had to split up, and then this other guy I
don't know comes into the room, and says, you know, I'll call
this guy and I'll call that guy, and who's in charge here, who's
taking charge of all this, and I thought, that guy, I'll smash his
head against the wall and throw him out the window, all these
people shouting and lining up and shoving everyone around,
and so I said to them, shouting, you know I screamed at them,
why don't you filthy bastards get out of here, and you freaking
scum and leave me and my sister alone I need to talk to her,
you freaking dirt, why don't you shove out of here, you freaking faggot dope addicts, get out of here, I screamed, oh God, I
screamed at them and I don't know what I'd have done if Miss
Bampton hadn't shown up just then and just walked in the door
and stood there, you know, just stood there like the Mother of
God and waited for the quiet.

Ten

Everyone whispers to me then, you know, about Miss Bampton, how she is Kathy's voice teacher, and how she used to sing at the Metropolitan Opera, and then I see, right, how she could be this huge star, because she just stands there in this vast tornado of a fur coat, and her hair piled up on her head, and a hundred necklaces around her whatchacallit, you know, bodice, and lace, you know, all this lace cascading down her front, and her eyes are flashing and taking in the room and, as though she were just standing there waiting for the applause; and this girl from Kathy's music school says, she's just like a mother to Kathy, and I thought you know, well, this is the first I've heard of it.

Miss Bampton did, Kathy thought, look something like her mother. Something about Miss Bampton's high cheekbones, something about the fineness of her nose, the delicacy of the nostrils, something about how close her eyes were to tears; and yet she was not an entirely satisfactory mother; she was too dazzling to be anything but distant, too extraordinary, too

much possessed by others and by all, however much she and
Kathy especially favored one another; and even more than all
the other reservations, Miss Bampton was too reserved, too
qualified, too much the teacher, too dedicated to the notion
that her charge earn praise and applause, too unwilling to give
unqualified love, love without condition, love without de-
mand, love without measure of her pupil's good behavior,
talent, skill, smile, or character.

Patrick was impressed with the thought that Miss Bampton
was the unique adult among the youngsters. She did not cry,
nor wail, nor curse; she did not sit on Kathy's bed.

Without much being said—save how do you feel, fine thank
you, I brought these for you—the young freaks and frantic
friends, hysterics and pillpoppers quietly drifted out of the
room and into the corridor. Her manner was formal, and
somewhat stiff. She brought flowers.

Eleven

Kathy Morris? Hello, good morning, I'm Dr. Cunnought. We met yesterday.

Yes.

She thought his briskness would save her life, and she was pleased to see how the cheerfulness of his greetings had shocked the last of the Bohemians lingering at the door.

This is Miss Bampton. She's my voice teacher.

How do you do?

And my brother Patty.

Patrick?

Yeah. Hi.

Cunnought observed that she introduced no one else, and so it seemed to him that Miss Bampton and Patrick should stay while he talked to Kathy. He asked Kathy whether she would like them to stay, and she said she would and all the others, friends and voyeurs, vanished quietly, well-rehearsed spear carriers. Miss Bampton, Kathy noticed, stepped upstage left, and Patrick sat on Kathy's bed.

Do you have any questions?

You're a neurosurgeon.

Yes.

What's going to happen?

What have you been told?

I have a tumor.

Yes?

And it has to be removed right away.

Yes.

What's going to happen?

Well, first of all, the results of the angiogram are just great.
We now know exactly why you have had the seizures you've
had. Lots of times, people will come into the hospital, having
had seizures, and we just won't know what to do about it. We
just don't know how to control them. We will give the patients
medicine, and they will have more seizures, and our hands will
be tied. There's nothing else we can do. In your case we know
exactly what it is. We know exactly why you have the seizures. We know exactly what needs to be done.

I have a tumor.

Yes, you have a tumor, but it is a benign tumor. It is absolutely, unequivocally not malignant. It's the kind of brain
tumor that can be totally removed, and it's a situation in which
you can be absolutely cured. It's even conceivable that you can
be out of the hospital in seven to ten days.

It seemed to Kathy that the doctor's thoughts were constantly moving, darting, scanning, considering, and reconsid-
ering. It seemed to her that he loved his work, and she wished
that he would sit with her now for a long while, until dark at
least, until it was time for her to go to sleep, and talk with her,
explain things to her, things of all kinds, in a long rambling

conversation about nothing in particular, but long and aimless and drowsy.

Or I could die.

Or you could die. In any serious surgery of this sort, there is a chance of dying; and, because your tumor is on the left side of your brain, where your speech center is, there is a chance that you could come through the operation but be unable to speak, or read and write, or unable to sing, or just unable to think. You could become a vegetable, or you could lose the use of an arm or a leg, or become paralyzed all over. Any of these things is possible. All kinds of bad things can happen. But I'm just sure this operation is going to go very well. The tumor is just there on the surface of your brain, and we can just peel it off, and you'll be out of here in a week. I've done a lot of these, and this one is just a piece of cake.

Kathy listened to him speak and could not believe him, and so she nurtured the thought that she was in a show and that this was going to be a difficult role. She cast about for the proper character to play, whether Helen Keller (too old) or Anne Frank (too melodramatic). She would have preferred a musical comedy—*Man of La Mancha,* or *Camelot.* She had never appeared in *My Fair Lady,* often wanted to, thought this might be her opportunity; yet not even that seemed quite appropriate. And then, every once in a while, from moment to moment, it occurred to her that this might be, or perhaps even was, real, and she commenced to cry, without quite noticing it, thinking that she might not be a singer at all. She hoped that he was a Republican, and that he spent a good deal of time hobnobbing with bankers and steel executives. She did not want a wishful thinker to be cutting her up.

When is this going to happen?

Well, I'm really not sure, but I hope it can be either next
Thursday or Friday.

But somebody told me it would be done on Wednesday.

Yes, I thought it would be, too, but we've had to reschedule
it.

Why?

I thought you were a private patient, so I scheduled you
originally on the private schedule. The ward schedule for the
operating room is just a different schedule, so I've put you on
that for Thursday or Friday.

But I don't want to be a ward patient.

There's no difference really, just a matter of scheduling. I
thought originally that you had some sort of insurance coverage, that's all, so I thought you would come under the
schedule for private patients. You're not covered, so you come
on the ward schedule, that's all.

So I'm not going to get the best care. I'm a ward patient,
after all.

No, no, no. Not at all. Everything is just the same, the
operating room, the nurses and the doctors, everything is absolutely all the same. It's nothing but an administrative kind of
paperwork.

Except the operation is postponed. Everyone said I needed it
right away, and now you hold it off because I cannot pay.

Well, right away, yes, but it's not an emergency. A few
days this way or that . . .

So how much would it cost?

I don't really . . .

How much?

Gosh, I don't . . .

How much?

The surgeon's fee is two thousand dollars, your room for a

week or two could be a thousand dollars, the anesthe-siologist . . .

Say fifteen thousand dollars.

Oh, it wouldn't be that much.

I'll get the money, that's all there is to that. I'm not going to be shunted off into the ward again to die.

There is absolutely . . .

This is, you know, said Patrick, fucking unfair.

Why?

Because, you know if we had the money, then you would operate on Kathy on Wednesday.

Medically, surgically, as far as her care is concerned, it does not make any difference at all whether it's on Wednesday or Friday.

If it doesn't make any difference to you, and it doesn't make any difference to the hospital, and it doesn't make any dif-ference medically, then they can reschedule it, because it makes a difference to Kathy. We'll sell our house.

What house?

We have this fucking house we'll sell.

No, I won't let you do that.

We'll sell the house.

No, I won't let you sell your house, absolutely not. You will get the very same care whether you are on one schedule or another, I absolutely guarantee it. I'll be here one way or another, I'll be taking care of you, absolutely. And all the other doctors and nurses are especially watching out for you, and you're going to be just fine.

Oh, shit, you know, if she's not okay, I don't know what I'll do.

I don't know what you're worried about, Patty. It's my problem, not yours.

Cunnought stiffened, thinking, No, that was a cruel thing to say, and untrue, too, for it would be Patrick's problem, and not hers at all if something went wrong in the operating room, if she died—or ended up needing someone to care for her the rest of her long life. It was the cruelest thing she could have said, and if she lived, lingering, confined to bed, unable to speak or move or godknowswhat, it was the sort of thing her brother would not ever be able to bring himself to forget.

Well, it's okay, she said, to a fresh trio of students who threw themselves unknowing into the midst of the scene. Everything will be okay. This is my doctor, Dr. Cunnought, and this is my brother, Patrick, and you know Miss Bampton. The doctor tells me I have a meningioma, a benign kind of tumor, and he will take it out, and it is, he says, a piece of cake. He says it's a piece of cake.

She's going to be just fine. She's going to do just very well indeed, absolutely unequivocally. Listen, I'm going to check back with you tomorrow, Kathy, but I want you to have my phone number in case you want to call me for any reason, absolutely anything at all. You won't be able to get hold of me, but I check in with my answering service all the time, and I'll get right back to you. My number's on this card, and Patrick, I want you to have one, too, and Miss Bampton, please call me for any reason at all, at absolutely any time.

She tried to say, before he went out the door, that he should let her die if she couldn't sing—that if, in the middle of the operation, it looked to him as though something had happened so that her speech center were somehow hurt, or whatever might happen, that she would not be able to sing again that he should just let her die.

It occurred to her that he might not really care about her singing—that he might say he cared, that he might care in some half-attentive way, but he did look to her a little bit like a man who lived in Westchester and played golf, a little boy who thought of women as people to come home to, who thought it was nice for women to have talents for singing or piano playing, weaving or water coloring but who knew, finally, that all that really mattered for a woman was to marry and have children—and for that, she thought he thought, all she would really need was half a mind.

   She thought it would be best if she could be alone. She knew how best to gather her wits if she were left alone; she was accustomed to dealing with a crisis on her own.

Twelve

And suddenly she felt a temper tantrum about to overtake her, and she was alarmed and powerless.

I've got to get out of here. Somebody's got to get me out of this.

You'll be all right. (Miss Bampton said.)

I really need to get out of here. I'm not going to lose my voice.

Your voice.

I'm a singer, you know. I'm a pretty good singer. I think I'd better get out of here, because if there's any threat to my voice, you know, I'd just as soon die as lose my voice.

Patrick had often wondered as he was growing up, what was real and what illusion and at what point and whether thinking made it so, and why now he thought this was unreal when, in truth, in fact, if his sister were ever to throw a temper tantrum, surely this was the right occasion. And yet, he could not quite see why this insistence on her voice, her singing, so what if she lost her voice as long as she lived? Who needs to sing? He hardly ever had the need himself, although he must concede, he valued the gift of speech, he enjoyed palaver and the odd moment of chewing the fat, chewing the rag, giving lift to the timeless prattle, he agreed that creative utterance was the uniquely human gift, the miracle of miracles, the arc-lit zinger that traced a course of consciousness through the seeming chaos of the neurons, the mind, whatever and wherever, this and that the unique power that gave articulation to the miracle of consciousness, from synapse to galaxy or god, and that without it human life was not quite human life, not fully so in any case, and he lied to his sister when he told her that it did not matter so long as she was alive, life itself was the greatest boon (no doubt of that; he told the truth in that precise instance), no matter if she lost her voice (although, in fact, of course she would not lose it), but even so she insisted no, that if she did not have her music, she wanted nothing and no one, she'd rather die, without her music she'd have nothing; but no, Patrick insisted, you'd have me, but no, she said, I want my music, cutting him again, I'm nothing without my voice.

You're alive without your voice!

I'm not alive without my voice.

First comes life, and then comes singing.

No, I am a singer first.

That's stupid, that's a stupid thing to say. No singer says that, not even the best that ever lived in all the world.

Well, I say it then, best or not, it doesn't matter. I wish I were a star, Patty, and very rich but it doesn't matter, none of that. A singer is just who I am, like you're a man, and if I'm not I won't be me, it doesn't matter if I'm rich and great, but if I can't sing in my life then I don't want to live.

Don't say that or you'll die and go to hell! Don't say that or I'll tear this place limb from limb I'll get you out of here! You

will not die! You promised me! Don't give me that! What!
You can't leave me! I'm not taking any more of this!

Quietly he heard the voice, Miss Bampton's, and thought it
was not real at all: You'll be fine, Kathy. It just depends upon
your attitude.

What do you know? his sister replied in a voice of terror that
he remembered well. It's my career that's been broken, not
yours. It's mine. How could you know?

And then Miss Bampton cried, believing, too, that it did not
so much matter whether her pupils became rich and famous so
long as the music that she taught them somehow informed their
lives. She remembered then the time that Kathy fell and cut her
foot, and she took her home and cared for her, and gave her
dinner and put her to bed. Miss Bampton had not been among
the most dazzling of the stars of the Metropolitan Opera, not
one in any case who is remembered as Ezio Pinza is, or Risë
Stevens, or Jan Peerce—all of whom sang with her at the Met
in all those years, almost twenty years, that she was a member
of the company, and yet she had had a splendid career until at
last she could no longer manage the soprano roles, and her life
was broken, too, with that cruel loss of powers that seems to
be the special destiny of singers and dancers, to remind us all
of the transitoriness of beautiful things, and she vanished from
the company to reappear again two years later in recital at
Carnegie Hall, appearing there for the first time not as a soprano, but as a mezzo-soprano, and treated more than cour-
teously by the critics for her courage in attempting to make the
difficult, almost impossible, change of voice. She sang a while
longer, giving concerts here and there, and then came at last to
teaching at Kathy's school and The Juilliard School, nourishing
herself still with music, with the sound of the voice—even

though it was no longer her own—the sounds of scores of voices, rich and strong and thin and harsh, knowing that the value of the music lay deep within, deep amid structures that had never been explored by any but musicians—not by poets or linguists or logicians or physicians, but only by those who sang and played and wandered in the barely discovered territory of harmony and dissonance, time and duration, pitch and pure relationship, recollection of single notes or silences.

And so she cried, believing that she had not instructed her pupil in the most elementary lesson, that it is not important for a singer to have a voice; and Kathy joined her, crying, too, and Patrick, too, all three of them cried.

Thirteen

Lose her voice! Lose her voice! Patrick heard the students cry and wondered why he heard no swell of music from the orchestra. Word went down the corridor and back again; the crowds pressed in the room. Some were moved, of course they were, and truly so; girls wept. One fell dizzy. Boys were tense, with frightened eyes. What was this? To lose her voice? To live or die was bad enough—but lose her voice? What next? What worse? To lose the use of arm or leg, go blind or stupid, live a slack-jawed life, comatose, a vegetable, to lie abed for forty years or fifty years, drooling and obscene, babbling, and laughing, and fouling the sheets, sent off somewhere to a state asylum with other freaks and wrecks and medical mistakes. Get on the phone! get on the phone! call the *Times* and call the *Post*! get help. find out. make noise. insist. bring in another doctor, we'll have a consultation. we want the best, spare no expense, get money, fast. by God, for all the drama of the scene it did seem, too, that after all it might be really real.

but this hardly seemed the time, with all the crowds around.
Jeremy wanted the kids to leave, or else for him to leave. You
ought to pay, the kids seemed to say with their contemptuous
glances: you have the house and the lawn and job, the bank
accounts, the suits, the haircut, the tennis racket, and the age.

And Abigail thought, but yes, he has a family of his own,
and no one said we're rich, we've had to work and save and
plan ahead, add, subtract, organize our funds and dole them
out, a little bit for drapes and something for upholstery, cal-
culating costs of eight highball glasses, snifters, wine glasses
for the white and red and other crystal, and able at last to
afford a child, now this, now suddenly a huge expense because
their niece had not thought, or was too much the artist, too
much Bohemian, too much contemptuous of such Middle-
Class concerns, to have bothered with insurance coverage for
herself, she was lucky, was this niece, that she was the first
disaster, when it was still possible and affordable for her Uncle
Jeremy to say yes, he'll pay, never mind, I'll take care of the
whole thing, and never mind the thanks.

A student messenger arrived: I've made a call to school, to
see if there's insurance.

No, there's no insurance.

All students have insurance.

No, there's no insurance.

How much will it cost?

Fifteen thousand dollars.

My God.

Fifteen thousand dollars.

Jesus.

Who says?

Someone asked the doctor.

Who asked the doctor?

How much?

Fifteen thousand dollars.

The sons of bitches.

Fucking ripoff.

No wonder the sons of bitches are so rich.

How much?

Fifteen thousand dollars.

Oh wow.

For the whole thing. Breakfast included.

Enter Mrs. Hornbeck, a teacher, talking.

I've brought you some opera magazines, Patrick heard Mrs. Hornbeck say, and a little radio so that you can listen to some music, dear, I was just mentioning your name an hour ago to Kajah Khan—do you remember?—who's going to have an audition for the Met—the Met! that's right—and can't make up her mind, you know, whether to go ahead now and have her audition or wait and study for two more years and have the audition then, because, you know, it will never do to have an audition and do very badly, for it is hard to have a second chance with the Met, or at least it's very hard indeed, if you've had first a first chance and then a second, ever in the world to get a third, and so I was saying to her . . .

I don't want to hear this, please.

What's that, dear?

I don't want to hear about an audition for the Met when I'm about to lose my voice.

Lose your voice? I hope not, dear.

The only thing you can do for me now is get me fifteen thousand dollars, to have an operation like a private patient instead of being put through this hellhole place like some kind of lower-class lace-curtain goddam nigger they get around to after they've taken out the garbage.

I'm not sure I . . .

I don't want to hear about your goddam Japanese singers on their scholarships going to the Met, don't you understand me? I'm right here. I'm a singer, too, and I'm right here, and I'm a good singer, too, what the hell is going on in this place, why won't someone help me, all I need is some goddam money just so I won't die.

Well, the school insurance doesn't exactly . . .

She was appalled by her behavior. She had not guessed what savagery she had within her. She had no idea she hated people so—not just blacks, but everyone; she was possessed with cutthroat rage for all the world; it made her tremble; and she was amazed how murderous she felt. She wondered who she was; she wondered where she had come from. She wished she could rid herself of this malign urgency, this foul language, these fits of terror; but, even as she wished to calm herself, she would be seized with confusion and a fit of rage again; her eyes would widen, and she would savage her own good wishes of herself. Patrick was silent now; he recognized his sister not at all, and he was even more profoundly scared.

Then shove the school insurance and give me money! Take some of the money you fling at all those goddam Japs and Chinks and godknows whatall they all are and give it to me, Kathy Morris, American all my life and goddam dying!

Don't get excited, dear. . . .

I *am* excited! I *am* excited! I wish you'd get excited—and you would if you half began to understand what's going on. What the hell is going on? You've lost all touch with the way it is. I think you've lost your mind!

Now, then . . .

Get out! Get out! Go fuck your Japs! Get out of here, my God, what's going on?

Mrs. Hornbeck, thought Patrick, was amazed, and wandered blindly from the room, an older woman, somewhat round, with a gentle disconcerted manner. She wandered to the corridor; Patrick took her arm without quite thinking and stopped with her there at the end of the hall before the window overlooking the Cathedral of St. John the Divine. You know, she said, the church was begun about 1911, and the choirmaster comes from Juilliard. He turned and walked with her the few short steps to the elevators, and she spoke affectionately of Bach and Britten even as the doors were closing.

I need to take a walk. Is there any place to walk in this bloody hellhole?

And she donned her robe, letting it rest loosely about her shoulders like a cape, and the crowd parted as she made her stately progress from the room, followed in a moment (*Exeunt omnes.*) by her entourage, and down the disinfected corridor toward the east.

She knew she played her role awkwardly; there had been no time to rehearse, and this was, in any case, a desperate improvisation, without any motive that she could imagine—a sudden flight to the stage, a seizure of theatrics, shifting without warning from dying princess to *La Bohème,* from *Youth Denied* to *Man of La Mancha,* a gesture from *My Fair Lady,* a sigh from *A Streetcar Named Desire,* a search from Sartre for the exit.

Words failed her.

Her fellow students were unfailingly generous in this group improvisation, as they accommodated the shifts in role on the part of the leading lady, and, as she swept along the corridor she could imagine the students variously costumed as harlequins and clowns, circus performers, Robin Hood's merry men, attendants at the court, Lords and Ladies, latter-day barons of industry,

Members of Parliament, Communist agitators, righteous cler-
gymen, the James brothers. They all felt at home at last on stage,
safe, secure in this world of more real reality, where no pretense
is made of certainty but all conviction is given over to the truth of
shifting passions, uncertain character, the fleeting, the merely
apparent, the momentary glimpse of the significant insight passing too quickly to grasp.

At the end of the corridor, she turned, and stood, and was
alarmed to discover that she could think of no speech to give, no
passage from a play, not even any single line of rallying cry,
indeed, no single word. She did not know who she was, and she
was overcome with a sudden rush of panic. She had lost herself
again and so, with widened eyes, horrified, she swept back
through the crowd and headed west.

Perhaps someone would be attracted by the noise, she
thought, and step forward to intervene, some benefactor, some
kind person to say, here! enough of this! be off with you,
children! give my little girl peace. come to me, my dear, there,
there, leave everything to me, never mind, no, no, you needn't
concern yourself about anything at all now, I'll see to everything, come, come, let me hold you, now, yes, go right ahead,
you needn't fear to cry, put your head here on my shoulder, go
ahead and cry my love, yes I love you, dear, my little girl,
there, there.

Or, if not that, then at least some sort of embrace, some firm
grasp, some control to stop the trembling, for now she had
entirely lost her sense of self-possession.

At the west end of the corridor, she turned again and faced
her entourage, the courtiers, and once again she had no
speech, no line, no word, no name to give, and now she
noticed the lack keenly, feeling somewhat embarrassed and
sensing a hotness to her face, a moisture at the corners of her

eyes. She set out one more time now, heading to the intersection of the corridors, standing for a moment at the trans-
verse, then turning left, heading south.

When she had been very young, when her mother had come
to stop her tantrums, and neither she nor her mother knew
quite what to do, she had been grateful for her mother's presence, and she wished now that she might find some conjuring
trick that would bring her mother to her, some special form of
misbehavior, some nasty word or ugly face, a shriek or cry or
choking sound, but when she turned to face back north along
the corridor she only saw the head nurse, red-faced, coming
through the crowd, perhaps to scream at her or knock her
down. The nurse stopped, hands on hips, and then changed her
tactics midway through an angry scowl, and with face con-
torted in an effort to become calm and sweet, said thickly,
Kathy, I think you ought to go back to your room.

No, thanks. I'm, you know, fine, said Kathy inexplicably,
you can go to hell—and the nurse careened abruptly back
along the corridor, calling out for orderlies and interns, residents and attendants.

The progress was resumed, northward now, its leading
character rendered desperate by her own behavior, her vision
blurring now, gait uncertain, stumbling up against and coming
off the wall, her followers wild-eyed once again, distraught
and stumbling, too, into one another: what can they do to me
now? the leading lady cried out, throw me out on the street?
what's the worst they'll do to me? give me back my clothes
and send me home? then let them go ahead! let them do it!

At last a speech; and it was met by cheers and loud applause. The students cried and sat and sprawled and leaned
against the walls and laughed and shouted out, right on! and
clapped and cheered and smiled.

Throw me out then! Throw me out!

Throw her out, the chant went up, throw her out, then, throw her out!

The residents and interns rounded the corner of the intersection at last, bringing with them orderlies, nurses, medical students, ambulatory patients and patients in wheelchairs, visitors, guards, and the Episcopal chaplain of the hospital.

One doctor seemed to be in charge. He stopped some several yards before the youthful company and waited for the silence. He stood his ground for several moments, saying nothing, sizing up the crowd. And when at last he simply said that visiting hours were over, the students moved with quick relief to find the elevators.

Abigail took her arm, then, and led her back to bed. She had nothing more to say, nor did the others have anything left to respond. Who was still there? She looked about the room and found her brother and her uncle and her aunt. She was surprised to see that they looked tired. She had gotten rid of all but these few hardy souls and these, too, she had savaged fiercely. She was given several pills at once—she knew not what—but she was grateful that they calmed her, and made the trembling in her hand and arm and on down along the right side of her body cease.

You know I had to hurt someone, she said.

Sure, her uncle Jeremy said, of course you did.

They sat in silence for a while longer, while Jeremy thought of nothing but the amber light that suffused the whole of the hospital, the amber light and light green walls in the rooms and halls, and men's room, too, the inescapability of the amber light and then he said that he thought they ought to leave, pleading hunger and Abigail's pregnancy as an afterthought, they would take Patrick too, who had forgotten to eat all that day, they said good night, exchanging stiff, cold hugs—and then just before they left Jeremy said that Kathy need not worry; he would pay for her operation—and she said, right, then I won't have to wait, I can have it right away, and he said right, and then he left with Abigail.

Patrick followed, after hesitating, unsure and seemingly confused, and then returning to the bed and holding his sister for several moments, hugging her and saying something easy about seeing her tomorrow, then he left, too.

Alone, then, and thinking for a time, she wished that someone would make love to her. She wished Jay would return, or one of the doctors, but preferably Jay, and that they would make love, that she might doze off and wake again to make love once again, and she and Jay would sleep and wake and they would make love so often that she would at last completely lose her mind, she would not be really there, and she would be alive. And as she went to sleep, she realized that she had been so self-involved that she had entirely forgotten to thank her uncle Jeremy for offering at last to pay the hit man.

She and Jay might go out, then, to have dinner at Three Sisters and listen to the music, and they would not speak of the child they had almost had, but they would feel at ease with one another and when they left he would hold her coat and care for her and take her arm like an old-fashioned husband and father.

She understood that Jay needed time alone; they all did, these musicians—many hours a day—when they would leave the world, whether out of love or misery, to search some other place for harmony or adventure. Jay lived among the warehouses down in Soho, three flights up a cold and filthy stairway to his loft, cold and bleak, with old stove and refrigerator, an alcove for a mattress, and a large, high-ceilinged room, tin-plated, painted white, plants hanging in front of the wall of windows—nothing else but drums, smooth and polished, tuned and buffed, quivering on their stands whenever one walked near them. Jay rose late every morning, drank coffee, watered plants, limbered up, ate little for lunch and then, just after midday, and through the early afternoon, he played his drums, without any other music in the room, the drums alone for several hours. And again at night, with friends, or if he had a job then at a jazz club, he played till early morning, lost entirely among the sounds.

If she had had a son, she would have read to him from the very first so that he would love the sound of language, the play of words, so that he would read stories, novels, poetry, medical texts, and history. If she had had a daughter, she would have encouraged her daughter to sing, or do any other thing, to read or to play baseball or swim, to be a movie star or senator, and she would try to stay alive herself, for that would be the greatest gift she could give her children, and they her, and she would tell her daughter not ever to have an abortion, and she prayed that she would not be struck down now for having done wrong herself.

Fourteen

She woke up early Sunday, woke up singing quietly and to herself, humming then a bit and singing once again, trying out a phrase or two and then a verse or chorus. She thought she might not ever sing again, and so she sang half a dozen of her favorite songs. She had a powerful and rich voice, and she could have been heard in the back of the hall without any trouble at all. Her voice had the color and complexity of an operatic voice.

Fifteen

Later on that Sunday morning, Alvin arrived. The sun was out. And the priest came by. She had a flower on her breakfast tray. Patrick read the sports section.

Then she sang while Alvin played guitar, and they recorded several songs on the tape recorder. I will tell of a hunter, she sang, whose life was undone; his arrow was loosed and it flew through the night, and the shaft found its mark. A Peter, Paul, and Mary song.

Sixteen

Later on that afternoon, Aunt Abigail and Uncle Jeremy came by again and said they had to be on their way back home to Delaware, that they would return later in the week when Kathy had her operation. But Kathy said, the operation may be tomorrow. Then we'll come right back, said Jeremy. The terror paralyzed her eyes again, the terror and the anger, and all three of them could see that she was about to present a reprise of the day before.

I can't believe this, that now just when I need you you're going to leave me.

Well, Kathy, you know I must get back. I have a job; I left things in a rush to come, and . . .

Of course you did, this is no average thing. Who do I have but you and Abigail and Patrick? I have no one else, and now you say you're leaving? When else did I ever need you the way I need you now? I know you have a job, I know you have a house. What do you have to do, mow your lawn? Take down the screens? There's more than jobs and houses, come up to say hello, how is it going, well, we guess we'll be back on our way to do our jobs. I need you and you're bugging off, well then I don't need you. And if I die, I want you to be sure of this: I won't miss you!

Listen, I can't believe . . .

I can't believe it either. You know I lived with your father, and I grew up with him, and I was around the house with him all the time, and in the end when he was dying and you took him home to care for him, I know exactly how you felt, he was a nuisance to you, and you were waiting for him to die, and now you're waiting for me to die too, because I'm a nuisance to you.

I can't believe . . .

Well then get out!

Okay, well there's nothing I can do.

Well then get out!

There's nothing I can say to help.

Then get out of here!

I have nothing to say to you.

And I don't have a thing to say to you.

I don't believe you can talk like this. Who do you think has said they'll take care of all the bills? That's how I think we can help you best, that's what we're able to do. I'm not going to melt into a puddle and disintegrate. If you want us to fall down and cry at your feet, you're asking for the wrong thing.

Look, I have nothing more to say to you.

And I have nothing more to say to you.

Then get out of here.

I'm going.

Get out!

I'm getting out of here.

Hey, Jeremy, she took hold of the sides of her bed and

shook it violently, astonishing and frightening her uncle with her power—you never cry. I've seen you with your cool, you never cry, now you listen to me. You never cried when your brother died, and you never cried when your father died, now I'm telling you, I'm going to make you cry, if I have to die to do it, I'm going to make you into a real person, you cool bastard, I'm going to make you cry!

I'm going—get out!—I don't believe—I know—how immature—how you felt—your behavior is—when your father died—Jesus Christ! You've got you're not to love me dying you're going I'm not going to feel to be manipulated something by your hysteria I'm going, I am, oh no you're not, to make you, no one's going to feel to tell me something how to feel. Maybe I have nothing we're all supposed to die to say this way to you but I don't believe it you don't I don't if I get out of this you don't alive I don't there's nothing more want to see you to say again shut up get out I'm leaving go.

I'm going.

Good.

I'm leaving.

Get out.

Goodbye.

Get out.

Come on, Abigail. (*Exeunt.*)

Seventeen

She put her robe around her shoulders, her feet into slippers, and looked out the window for a time at the Cathedral. She composed the flowers on the windowsill, lingering there, plucking daffodils from one bouquet and placing them in another, exchanging rosemary for thyme on the bedside table, stacking the books neatly in pyramidal fashion, largest on the bottom, smallest on the top, then rearranging the stack to bury the book on dying at the bottom. She picked up the opera magazines that had fallen to the floor, and got back into bed, propped herself up grandly (with two extra pillows borrowed from the empty neighboring bed), and commenced to read every single word, beginning with the title of the magazine, the first advertisement, large print and small, THE EXCEDRIN HEADACHE. IT COMES IN ALL SIZES (read and follow label directions) and then, on the next page FINALLY, VANTAGE LONGS, and there the masthead, the names of all the editors, vice president and publisher, managing editor, associate editors, assistant editors, editorial assistants, correspondents, advertising director, please direct SUBSCRIP-TION CORRESPONDENCE, order changes of address, etc. . . . allow six weeks' advance notice, and then she read the table of contents, article and author, the letters to the editor, and then, at last, the lead article in the issue, taking care to read the head and subhead, noting each letter carefully, the body type, page number, issue date, hairline rule.

Eighteen

Cunnought entered with his usual buoyant boyish cheer, an enthusiastic hello, bright-eyed smile, springing step, how are you?

Fine, thanks.

Any questions?

No, not now.

Well, it looks as though we're going to be able to open up the ward schedule and get you into the operating room right away, first thing tomorrow morning.

Tomorrow?

Wouldn't that be great?

I thought it would be Wednesday.

Well now we have an opening in the schedule, and you and I can take it tomorrow morning. I thought you'd like that.

Yes, I would.

So would I.

What's going to happen?

In the morning, the nurses will bring you downstairs on the cart to an anteroom, and I'll see you there for a minute. And then I'll have to go and make sure everything is all set in the operating room. And then the nurses will bring you in, and I'll be there, you'll be awake, and you'll have a chance to see the operating room. It's nothing much, just a room with a big light, just the sort of thing you've seen on television. And then we'll put you to sleep with nitrous oxide—that's laughing gas—you may even have had it at your dentist's from time to time. We'll give you a little more than he does, and it will put you to sleep. We'll do the operation. It will take perhaps four hours; and then we'll wake you up and take you down to the recovery room. You'll spend the night in the recovery room, and then you'll be back up here.

You'll shave my head?

Oh, yes.

How much?

Well, we might as well shave it all, so it will grow out evenly.

You're not going to operate on my whole head?

No, no, no.

Then couldn't you just shave a little bit?

Sure, if you would rather. I'll just shave—well, I'll shave one side, how's that? We like to be sure we don't have any hair in the operating field, because we have to be certain that where we work is absolutely sterile.

Right.

So just one side.

Thank you. I wish you'd talk to me a little more.

What would you like to know?

There's nothing I want to know. I just wish you wouldn't leave.

Well, we both need our rest.

I know. What do you do on weekends?

If I'm off duty, and if I have the time, I go kayaking. And when I have a vacation, I love to take a canoe, and go down the Allagash River in Maine, go down the white water, spend some days there in the woods, camping out and getting up early in the morning to go down the white water.

I usually sing. For the past few years, to help pay my way through school, I have a gig on Saturday nights. I'll usually have a group, a drummer, say, and a piano and a sax, let's say, and we'll do some numbers. Not bigtime nightclubs, just little ones, you know, but they're dark, with candles here and there, or little lights, small tables, and very dark, I like it when it's dark, and you hear the voices a little bit, murmuring, and the glasses, the sound of ice cubes, or the snap of cigarette lighters, and then you know you have it when you hear no sound at all, not any sound but the music, and then you know you've got it together, and then you really sing, and that's the best. I need to sing, you know.

Yes, he thought, she may well need to sing, and he hoped she would. The notion of saving a singer appealed to him profoundly. But even so, he could not repress the thought that he wished for her first simply to survive. It would be a fine thing for her to be able to sing, but he wished at least she might be able to live, to marry and to have children, to keep house and engage in idle conversation.

I would like to hear you sing sometime, he said.

Would you kiss me?

Yes. Just as soon as the operation is over, and we all feel like celebrating.

Okay, then.

I'll see you in the morning.

Sleep well.

Good night.

Nineteen

Cunnought recalled that night, as he drove back across the bridge, having read somewhere as a child of a great New York neurosurgeon—his name had long since disappeared—who was asked what his most exciting time had been. The neurosurgeon replied at once that it had been the time he operated on the ulnar nerve of a virtuoso violinist, that nerve that passes through the ulnar bone and is called the violinist's nerve because it controls the fine coordinated movements of the hand. And Cunnought recalled having operated on Cynthia Carr, a young woman, Kathy's age, who several years before had had a malignant tumor that Cunnought removed. After the operation, some few months later, Cunnought attended Cynthia Carr's recital at the Union Theological Seminary and thought, as he listened, that he was the only one who knew how astonishing it was that this voice sang that night, how miraculous that the words and music had survived intact that violated brain, assaulted first by tumor and then by knife, and how, if not for him, as he alone well knew, she would not be singing there that night. And then he thought, too, of how she had written him from London a year or so after that recital, telling him of the recurrence of symptoms, and how he had calculated at once that he would not have the pleasure of hearing her sing again. He carried her letter in his wallet; it was the only memento of his trade that he indulged himself by keeping. He was impressed by song, by singers, and by singing. He could not sing at all himself, not even "Happy Birthday." That inability betrayed the only neurological deficit he had—so far as he knew. He had a tape of Cynthia Carr's recital at Union Theological Seminary, but he had not played it since she died.

Twenty

And when she was at last alone, and it was dark, long after
dinner, and she had tired of neatening the flowers, the nurse
left her finally with two small sleeping pills and a glass of
water. She went to the bathroom then and came back to her
bed, to the bedside phone, and tried to call her friend Jay. He
did not answer, and she imagined he must be out playing a gig
at Stryker's, and so she went to the bathroom again and then,
when she returned, she rearranged her flowers, tidied up her
books, went to the bathroom, and rearranged the flowers. She
moved the plant from her bedside table to the windowsill,
tidied up her magazines, went to the bathroom and came back
to bed, and took the sleeping pills, went to the bathroom, came
back to her bed, took off her robe, lay down, and closed her
eyes.

I saw my mother then, and I talked to her. I told her I was
afraid. I was very calm, but I was afraid, and she said to me,
it's not time for you yet, and I went to sleep with her, and as I
went to sleep, she talked to me, and held me and told me it's
not time.

PART TWO

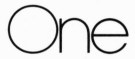One

He always woke up early, Cunnought recalled, when he had a
football game to play at Haverford, and he loved the early
morning hours; he loved to get up just a little earlier than his
customary hour and feel the edge it gave him, the fluttering of
nervous energy, the keen sense of the early morning light, the
chilliness that reminded him of his flesh, the sense that he was
aware of the stakes of the day even while others slept. He
loved the quiet of the house; he loved the coldness of the
bathroom floor, the shower, the coolness of his white shirt,
sound of the heels of his loafers on the bare wood floor, the
terrible coldness of the car, the fast drive, quick turns at the
corners, pressing closer to the brink of skidding on the ice,
pumping on the brakes, the precision of the turn, keeping
exactly to the millimeter within the traffic lane across the
George Washington Bridge, ten miles above the speed limit.
He eased back and coasted then, his adrenalin up to proper
levels, on call as needed, he stayed just on the edge of en-
thusiasm, saving his reserves.

The surgeons' locker room at St. Luke's was not merely like
the locker room of a football team; it was a club room for
nothing but the quarterbacks and left halfbacks, nothing but
legends in their own times. Cunnought's locker Number 25
was just next to that of one of the great cervical spine surgeons
of New York, one of the few great cervical spine surgeons, for
that matter, of the world; and farther down the row of lockers
were some of the members of the open heart surgery team, one
of the great open heart teams anywhere. And among these stars
of the operating theater, only the neurosurgeon worked alone.
He had the help of nurses and anesthesiologists and a resident
physician, to be sure; but for the essence of the operation, he
was not a team player; he was alone.

New York Hospital had several neurosurgeons; Bellevue
had Ransohoff and a couple of others; St. Barnabas once
starred Irving Cooper; but in all Manhattan, there were no
more than two or three score neurosurgeons, and they knew
one another well, by reputation and by handshake, by cocktail
party chatter and by sitting down after dinner to watch the slide
shows of one another's recent successes and failures. What
would you have done here? We attempted a suboccipital ex-
ploration. At the Neurological Institute Lester Mount would
spend several hours before his operations studying the X-rays,
planning his strategy, so that when he got onto the sterile field,
he would have no surprises.

Cunnought stripped to his undershorts, put on loose, light-
green drawstring trousers, loose, light-green shirt, sterile hat
and mask, and a pair of clogs—white, for the operating room,
and speckled with blood.

He considered how he had always been impressed with himself as he went into an exam. Beforehand, he might be anxious
and on edge and upset that he had not studied enough; but, as

he walked into the examining room, the fear would dissolve; he was buoyed up and looked forward to the event, exhilarated and sure he would never forget it.

She was awakened—tenderly, she thought—at six o'clock on Monday morning, by a nurse so lividly black as to be momentarily frightening. She asked the nurse how much time she had, and the nurse said that they wanted her at six thirty, and she thought half an hour is a long time to wait. She thought that she was ready, and she thought now she could make it if only they would hurry up and do it. The nurse gave her two small pills, and she turned over, and the nurse gave her an injection. She wanted to go to the bathroom then, and she got out of bed, and the nurse told her to put on her slippers, but she did not want to put them on. It seemed a small thing, to do what she wished about the slippers, but the nurse chased her to the bathroom with the slippers.

When she returned to the bed, she took off her pajamas and put on a white gown, so white she thought she might get married. Her hands were numb, and her head was entranced, and she thought she felt much too fine to have a brain tumor, but she was cold, and soon enough she felt nothing at all but the cold.

Hurry up, she thought.

Do it.

Let's get it over with. Hurry up.

The nurse helped her then onto the cold steel cart, and they went down the hall, and she was looking at the nurses and the orderlies, but this was the night shift still, and she didn't know these people, and she missed the ones who came on in the morning. She was very cold, and she thought of Jay, and she wondered why he wasn't there to care for her. She thought she would ask to make one last call, and get off the cart and call him from a pay phone in the hall: hello, Jay, calling you from corridor to the electric chair, just to say hello, you know, just to see how you are this morning; don't want you to worry about a thing, because everyone tells me that it's no big deal. Jay thinks he looks like Alfred E. Neumann, but he doesn't, not at all; he has long curly hair, and he wears blue turtlenecks most of the time.

She was very cold; thinking hurry up now.

Downstairs she saw the anesthesiologist in the large room where all the patients wait, lying on their carts, waiting for the operating room to be ready for them, and her mouth was dry, and she wanted to tell him that the last time she had this feeling was when she had her tonsils out.

Let's do it.

And then Dr. Cunnought came by, but she was very sleepy, and told him that the reason was that then she became an alto for a while, and he said when was that, and she said when I had my tonsils out, you know, I never should have had my tonsils out, because then I lost my voice, but he just smiled and said that she would be fine, but she knew she never should have had her tonsils out, and she meant to say if I can't sing don't let me live, but all she thought to say was, let's go I'm ready, and the next thing that she knew she was in the operating room, where she saw the overhead stainless steel ceiling light, and the walls were all of light green tile, and all along one wall were machines and X-ray viewing boxes, and all along another were medicines in a cabinet, and all along the third was the spectator's window, and all along the fourth wall were the windows and the sunlight and the wonderful sky, and just the very top of the Cathedral of St. John the Divine, and that was good, and then she twisted around and looked down at the floor, and the floor was made of tiny tiles, all colored dark

maroon, or a brownish shade of maroon—so that they
wouldn't show the blood—and so she turned over on her back
again and thought that she might faint.

Cunnought came in the room then and said good morning to
Anne, the nurse who was setting out her instruments, and to
Tsing, the anesthesiologist; to Luddy, the resident who would
assist him; and to several others who assisted the assistants.
They all helped move the cart over next to the operating table,
and held it there, helping Kathy ease over from the cart onto
the table. (What other sacrificial victim has to climb up on the
altar?)

Tsing and his assistants—suddenly now he had four people
there to help him—took her over now, and Cunnought stepped
aside and left her to the ministrations of the anesthesiologist,
who had her—too soon!—asleep and gone; just before she
went, she whispered, Hurry up, and then the doctors and nurses
were all over her with intravenous needles, blood pressure
gauges, hookups for dextrose solution, blood transfusion, and
tubes thrust down her throat to do her breathing for her. The
technology had hold of her; the Datascope 850 tracked her
heartbeat on its screen, and the Ventilator puffed up its rubber
lung and breathed for her, and she was gone, and, as far as she
will ever know, she was completely dreamless, cast utterly
into a void, dark and absolutely timeless, a place past all
sensation, even while all vital signs remain acute, a place
created for her by nitrous oxide, sodium pentathol, the strong
narcotic sublimaze, and just enough curare to keep her motionless, paralyzed for the next few hours.

She was astonishingly naked, and, of course, vulnerable,
suddenly deprived of sheet and gown and laid out on the hard
steel table equipped with gears and crankshafts for making
adjustments of level, position, orientation, and everyone in the

room was abruptly silent—silent out of respect—and hushed
and awed as well by the beauty of this young girl and the
violent care about to be visited upon her defenseless—and at
the moment, indeed, it seemed, sacred, almost divine—body,
this fragile vessel of life—such thoughts as these hastened
from the room by rude thoughts of mastery, sadistic rites,
bondage games, and domination, and then affection, too, and
mere caring. Then she was covered with a sheet.

Cunnought took her head matter-of-factly in his hand, and
with his other hand yanked the head cushion from the table and
threw it to the floor. This specimen that he held in his left
hand, this piece of bone filled with neurons, required twisting
to the right, and though he seemed to meet with some resis-
tance because of all the tubes that went down its throat, he
turned the head and cranked the table to elevate the shoulders.
Tsing appeared to be concerned that Cunnought would pull out
all his tubes and needles, and Anne stopped setting out her
instruments to watch the doctor's rudeness, and then at last,
having placed the head where it best suited him, he secured the
gears and cranks and reached then for a small pillow that he
placed with care under Kathy's head, brushing back a strand of
her hair as he did so.

He reached then for a small high table set on casters next to
him. Set out upon a sterile white towel were soap and water, a
straight razor, and an electric shaver. With the shaver first, he
sheared the left side of her head, precisely one half as he had
promised her, precisely down the midline. He then put on a
pair of rubber gloves and laid on soap and water unsparingly,
scrubbing the head's left hemisphere under which the tumor
lay, scrubbing for several minutes as the first of several steps
in preparing an absolutely sterile field for his operation, and
scrubbing, too, to feel the movement and the warmth in his

shoulders and his arms, to move his fingers, to get in touch
again with the manner of his hands, to feel the tips of his
fingers move along the ridges and gulleys of this unique
cranium, to become acquainted with the swellings, the crests,
and the all but imperceptible crevices.

Then, with a straight razor, he shaved the head, quickly and
without hesitation, and without inflicting the smallest cut or
nick, sure of himself and feeling good, acutely in touch with
all his nerves and muscles, with the others in the room, the
light outside, in complete control, eager now to move ahead,
beginning now to be suffused with that sense of peace, the
sense of being all alone and absolutely sure, as though soaring,
that sense that comes in the operating room of being stunningly
alive and in control of life.

He felt the smooth shaven head now, and then reached for
the gauze sponges, soaked them in an antiseptic solution of an
ugly reddish brown, and scrubbed the head carefully with this
vile staining liquid. Once again he felt the contours of the
head, ran his fingers very lightly over the skin, coming to rest
delicately and nonchalantly down below the midline, toward
the left ear, on a mound about the size of the palm of his hand,
and he gazed up at the X-rays taped to the window, where he
could see, against the vault of the Cathedral across the street,
the blush of the tumor inside the translucent bone, and he
considered it for several moments before he took the sterile pin
from the table and outlined with a deep scratch in the flesh just
where he would make his incision, and, along the line of the
mark, he applied with a Q-tip a beautiful iridescent stain of
methalene blue.

He stepped back and touched nothing else. He removed his
gloves and glanced around the room to note that Anne and
Tsing were ready; just behind him Luddy stood, having al-

ready scrubbed, donning now the overgown with the help of a
young blonde nurse named Karen. Two orderlies stood by
him, and Cunnought said, you can go ahead and set up now,
I'm going to scrub.

As Cunnought left the room, the orderlies brought up a
rectangular metal table with tall stilt legs and moved it in to
straddle the massive table on which the patient lay. Over this
went a large light-green sterile cloth so that the patient was
covered at once as though by a soft catafalque. The head
emerged from one end of this catafalque, and there the surgeon
would stand with his assistant Luddy. To his left, on the side
with the medicine cabinets, was a control console on wheels, a
movable set of dials and knobs, viewing screens and reg-
ulators, that sustained and monitored the specimen that lay
upon the operating table. To the right, in front of the windows,
was Anne. She moved up her own set of several tables draped
with sterile green cloths on which she had put out her array of
clips and knives, forceps and elevators. She took several large
trays of instruments and mounted several steps to a jerry-built
summit made of half a dozen small steel platforms. She put her
trays of instruments out upon the sterile cloth-covered straddle
table, and thus she was prepared, with the most often used
instruments directly in front of her on the table just above the
patient's head, and with reserves of instruments several steps
down behind her, the mallets and spreaders, steel drills,
syringes, sterile water, sponges, the solid state electrocoagulator and the suckers. The sucker, or suction tube,
efficiently removes any blood from the field of operation—and
removes, too, any other unwanted detritus, any water, any
abscess, any damaged brain. (How do you tell good brain from
bad brain? The bad brain goes up the sucker.) The electrocoagulator stanches the bleeding of the small vessels by pass-

ing a tiny electric current through the vessel and cooking it closed, producing a pleasant, faintly sweet scent. With these two devices, the surgeon controls the bleeding, and, with the control of bleeding holds on to life and affords himself the leisure to explore.

Marshall McLuhan once had a meningioma removed by a surgeon who was so meticulous that the operation lasted for nineteen hours. The surgeon stayed on his feet at the table all that time while nurses and assistants and anesthesiologists were replaced in several shifts. Among the tubes that are inserted down the patient's throat are the nasogastric tube that goes right down within the stomach, and the esophageostethoscope that goes into the esophagus, close up to the heart, so that the anesthesiologist—by plugging an earpiece in his ear—can keep acute track of the patient's heartbeat. Weary in the early morning, the anesthesiologist connected yet another unit of blood—this time not to the intravenous line but to the nasogastric tube—and filled McLuhan's stomach with blood that came back up the esophageostethoscope. The surgeon looked up and momentarily thought that the anesthesiologist was hemorrhaging out both ears; Cunnought returned, with his newly scrubbed hands held, fingers extended up, before his chest. Karen gave him a towel, and he looked about the room once more. To Anne he said, do we have someone else ready to take over when you fall? Karen helped him into his light-green gown and placed upon his head the halo to which his own little headlight was attached. He shunned the large Zeiss microscope on its elaborate mounts and asked instead that the eyeglasses equipped with magnifying lenses be ready for him. He was helped into two pairs of gloves, one size seven and a half, one size eight, to make him doubly safe against some pin-sized hole that might break the sterile procedure and sow

fatal infection inside the head he was about to enter. For a
moment, as the surgeon stands back from the operating table,
as the last of the light-green sterile drapes are affixed to the
tables, all but entirely enshrouding the patient—and all that is
left for the surgeon to see is that field of green and that delicate
half-crown of flesh marked with its line of iridescent blue—the
room is quiet and lovely, transfused with the soft blue light
that comes through the window, and it is at that moment that
the surgeon seems most like a priest, so clean and soft, with
his delicate cream-colored gloves held lightly before him, and
he seems smooth and eager, clean and kind; at that moment the
ceremony and the priest are touched with a sacredness and
purity that is unspeakably poignant. The surgeon prolongs the
moment, waiting for instinct and training, will and calling,
caution and exhilaration to draw him to the table to cut the
flesh and bone.

He steps forward quickly, asking for a suture, and sews a
light-green towel directly to the scalp above the line destined
for the incision, another below the place that he will open up
the flap of skin, one to each side of his approach, then covers it
all with a transparent plastic sheet that adheres both to towels
and skin, then takes from Anne the syringe and injects here
and there, along the methalene blue line, a solution of epi-
nephrine that will retard the bleeding.

Knife.

He takes the inoffensive little piece of steel that looks as
though it were meant for soap carving or other children's craft,
with a blade no larger than his little finger's nail, a flat,
aluminum handle the length of a fountain pen. He is breathing
freely now, and cannot prevent himself from rising to his
tiptoes from time to time. He is alert. His eyes are quick. His
fingertips so sensitive to the touch as to feel themselves to be

the very edge of the blade, and he is high, he is blithe, he is exuberant, he is merry, and he quivers for an instant before he cuts, and cuts once more, keenly along the glowing line, in a long and beautiful, swooning arc rich in vigorous, quick blood, flowing thickly, like hot blackstrap molasses and seeming not at all frightening but rather exciting and nourishing, rousing urges of hunger and thirst.

With sponge and sucker, Luddy cleared the field of blood, and Cunnought retraced the blade's path with his cooker, his electrocoagulator, to close off all small bleeders. In this area of the scalp, he would come across no major veins, no arteries; later on he would need to take care not to cauterize any major vessels and thus disturb the necessary blood supply to the brain. Having made his opening in the scalp, Cunnought handed the knife to Luddy, to give the resident some experience of making this surgical approach.

You cut, he said, I'll cook.

A loudspeaker on the wall commenced to broadcast music softly; the radio was tuned to a station specializing in religious music. A hymn becalmed the room. Would someone, Cunnought asked quietly without looking up, change the station and get some music for us? The patient can't hear this anyway.

In the womb of the human female, the fertilized egg divides and grows into two connected spheres of cells. At the point at which the two spheres touch, the point of contact thickens. By the eighteenth day of pregnancy, the thickening has become a neural groove. The forward end of this groove thickens, too, and although the fetus is only one and a half millimeters long, swellings commence to appear that foretoken eyes, ears, and nose. The neural groove grows deeper, and the walls on either side rise up like the sides of a canyon and then, at the top, they touch, close over and seal shut. By the twenty-fifth day of pregnancy, a completed neural tube extends the length—all of five millimeters—of the embryo.

At the head of the neural tube of the twenty-five-day-old embryo, appear three swellings that correspond to the three swellings of the earliest of vertebrate brains—the hindbrain, little more than a thickening of the spinal cord, that is associated in the earliest vertebrates with the detection of vibration, equilibrium, and balance; the midbrain, associated with vision; and the forebrain, the farthest forward, associated in rudimentary brains with smell.

Soon, by the time the embryo is thirteen millimeters in length, the brain will have begun to show its five ultimate, distinctive features: the hindbrain, the midbrain, the thalamic region, and then the great swelling mushroom cap of the cerebrum that is divided into the left and right hemispheres. By the fifth month, these two hemispheres of the cerebrum will have begun to assume their densely packed aspect; more and more neurons will be added, and the cerebral surface, the cortex, will fold in and out on itself to provide the maximum possible surface for the gray matter. It is the gray matter that seems to be the distinctive working stuff of the brain cells, and the cortex is only as thick as an orange peel. Underneath that wrinkled layer is the white matter which derives its color from the heavy massing of axons that connect all the cells up on the cortical surface. In the nine months that the fetus grows in its mother's womb, an average of more than twenty thousand neurons will be formed in its brain each minute.

They went down through skin and flesh, through muscle down to bone, and, having cut a large and sleek hyperbolic curve, peeled back the flap to reveal the skull. The flap of skin and muscle is then edged with small, self-adhering Michel clamps—laid back, and forgotten. Vestiges of flesh are scraped away from the skull, and then the bone is flushed with water, sponge-dried and gleaming.

"It is not possible," Galen said, "to find a method of opening the skull which is devoid of danger and which can be done rapidly." Galen's recommended method consisted of making many small holes around the area of bone to be removed. The holes were made with a trephine, a sharply pointed perforator, and then the bone between the holes was cut with a chisel and mallet. Cunnought used an electric drill to make his burr holes. He put the drill together himself, checking the bit and other fittings as he did. The operator must press heavily to drill through the bone: this bone is rugged stuff, both hard and resilient; but the operator must not lean on the drill with all his weight. Although the drill stops automatically once it has pierced through the bone, the surgeon must be careful not to push the drill bit on into the skull, on into the brain. Having made the first burr hole, Cunnought gave the drill to Luddy, showing him two more places to drill holes—and remember this, the surgeon informed the young resident, to assuage his apprehensiveness, the first principle of neurosurgery is this: when you make a mistake, never say oops.

Several years ago at another hospital, Cunnought was on duty when a cop was brought in with a gunshot wound in his head. The police surgeon asked if he could scrub in on the case, and Cunnought said of course. Up in the operating room, Cunnought asked for the air drill, and it was handed to him piece by piece for him to put together, and he realized then he had no idea how to assemble the drill. This damned drill, he said, it never works; let me have the hand drill. Good God, old man—(it was the voice of Dr. Pool from the Neurological

Institute, ten years before, when Cunnought performed an
operation in the presence of that great man who was known for
the simplicity and directness of his surgical technique)—good
God! what are you doing? Where did you learn to do that?
Why all these burr holes? You really didn't read my book, did
you?

This is an ancient craft, the practice of surgery upon the
skull, and it is still, as it has been in tradition, an ardent
confrontation of art and science and utter ignorance, of
miraculous technology, of precision and sophistication, and
brutal bloodiness, of intelligence and savagery, of keenness
and clumsiness, of extreme control and luck and awful chance.
Some 400 ancient trephined skulls, said Cunnought, rest in the
Warren Museum of the Harvard Medical School, remnants of
a surgery practiced even before the four-thousand-year-old
Egyptian papyri first record any surgical procedure. These
skulls have been opened up by intention, by design. Cocaine,
derived from coca leaves, may have been the anesthetic; the
patients felt no pain. Their skulls were opened up by Galen's
technique, or, upon occasion, by rougher practice—by scrap-
ing, by cross-cutting with a sharpened piece of stone. Of these
400 skulls, a full 250 show the signs of postoperative bone
growth: 250 of these 400 survived the operation, an astonishing survival rate, a most respectable survival rate.

Many of these operations were performed on heads that had
been bashed or cudgeled, crushed or fractured, the result of
accidents or mayhem. Some of the ancient skulls—from the
burial grounds of Inca fortresses in the mountains of Peru—
were cracked in battle.

But some of the skulls show no sign of traumatic wound,
and in these cases, the operation may have been performed as a
religious or thaumaturgic rite to release the evil spirits that

seemed to cause epilepsy. Some of the ancient operations may even have cured cases of epilepsy. Some may have relieved cases of depressed skull fractures and sinus infections.

The surgeon hopes, when he makes his burr holes, that he will feel no pressure welling up from within the hole, no pressing outward of hemorrhage, say, of abscess or of inflamed brain. The anesthesiologist will have given the patient Mannitol, a drug that will cause the brain to subside somewhat, to shrink, to make some room within the skull in which the surgeon can move about. Cunnought once performed an emergency operation at which several agents of the CIA attended in the operating room, asking Cunnought from time to time whether the patient would revive, what chances the patient had of living. Cunnought found with the drilling of his first burr hole a violently swollen brain. The patient had been poisoned.

On this morning, the burr holes were clean and fine and, flushed with water, looked very promising. Just beneath the skull is the brain's last defense, a thin lining of what appears to be translucent gristle: the dura mater. Into the first burr hole, Cunnought slipped a Freer elevator, a miniature, stainless steel, flat-bladed spade, in along the top of the dura, between the dura and the skull, making certain that the two were not adhering to one another. Then he took the air drill once again, replaced the drill bit with a small fluted steel blade. With this, rather than with mallet and chisel, he connected his three burr holes and popped out the small round disk of bone.

The brain beats. Just as the heart beats, so does the brain, pulsing in all its vessels with the rhythm of the heart. Cunnought nips the dura, with a small flick of an incision and then once again, using his Freer elevator, he puts the flat wedge of steel just beneath the dura, places his knife point precisely atop the elevator, and quickly slices through the dura, keeping knife away from brain with the elevator, opening up the dura, laying it back upon the skull, opening up the naked, pulsing brain, and it is at once a stunning and an ordinary thing. It is wholly defenseless. It has no feeling whatsoever. The anesthetic eliminated any sensation of pain when the knife cut through skin and muscle, but the brain has no sensory nerves at all, nothing to warn it of this intrusion—because, if an invader has come this far, any warning is, in any case, too late. The brain is an unprepossessing thing, as though it would protect itself in this ultimate state of vulnerability by a camouflage of modesty. Aristotle was so unimpressed by its appearance that he concluded the brain was merely a cooling system for the spectacular heart.

The brain is of a size that would fit comfortably within the palms of two hands. It is pinkish-gray in color—pink because of all the blood vessels that course through it, and gray because of the neurons, packed in folds and ridges, that are its extraordinary element. It weighs, Cunnought said, about forty-five or fifty ounces, and it feels somewhat like jello. It is very smooth and soft and compact, and it often frightens those who come for the first time to trespass.

Cunnought paused and stepped back from the table to ask for his magnifying glasses. These glasses are made of an ordinary horn-rimmed frame and two large barrel-set magnifying lenses like those that a jeweler uses. Karen helped Cunnought put them on, and then she fastened a strap at the back of his head to hold them in place. With the glasses on, Cunnought resembled a cross-eyed, myopic, slightly crazed bombmaker. He looked at his own hands to make certain that the lenses were properly adjusted. How much, asked Anne, do those glasses magnify? Three times, said Cunnought (pause): if you have 20/20 vision to start with. He stripped off his top pair of gloves—they were flecked with blood—and put on a new pair.

Oh, it looks good, the surgeon says, this looks really good, it looks just fine, everything is really fine.

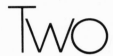

Two

As Cunnought descended into the brain before him, he entered a place that had, for him, some familiar features, some regions that he recognized, where he had been before. He knew the safe places and the dangerous ones, the resting spots, the areas he had to hurry past, where he had to go slowly and with care. He knew that at one summit or fissure, the great Harvey Cushing had run into trouble; elsewhere, he had seen a sudden eruption of blood, had seen a man paralyzed in an instant; at another spot, he had seen a man bleed to death, as he stood watching.

Some of these shoals and ledges and other natural wonders had been named by physicians centuries ago, by those conversant in Latin who discovered the pons—a structure that looks like a bridge over a chasm—and the hippocampus, which looks like a miniature, jeweled seahorse. Some places were claimed by the great nineteenth-century explorers who announced that they had found the temple of reason, and named these areas of the inscape for themselves: Broca's area, and Wernicke's area, ranges of sulci and gyri just above the Sylvian fissure.

It is in these regions that Cunnought loves to travel, where he loses consciousness of the world above, of his daily rounds, even of the room in which he performs, and he descends to a place that has its own adventures and dangers, its own myth and history, and its traces of other explorers whose presence Cunnought can still sense among the features of the place.

He descends near the fissure of Rolando, down along the smooth ledge of the temporal lobe, along the palisade of a silent area. No one knows just what might transpire here. Electrical probes find no answering response along these ridges.

Far below is the base of the brain, the brain stem that thickens out from the spine—the most forbidden territory, where one small misstep plunges into death. Nothing unfathomable occurs there; all is brutally simple. The hindbrain has three recognizable features, all staked out some centuries ago by medieval physicians: the medulla oblongata, a thick stalk of a thing, a stalactite; then the pons, the bridge that connects the medulla to the upper reaches of the brain; and the cerebellum, the twin spheres separated by a deep ravine that courses on up through the midbrain and the forebrain, cutting the cerebrum into two vast hemispheres.

Down in the region of the hindbrain, if one tugs on the medulla, the abrupt silence is shocking; it is the sound of someone having suddenly ceased breathing. Dread wells up in the silence; unseen forces are present; the quietness of cold-blooded animals pervades the place; creatures from another age prowl about these levels. Then, when the medulla is released, the breathing resumes. It is a terrific phenomenon—to tug on the thing and let it go and hear the silence, then the breathing, the silence once again, and then the breathing. A small boy could play with this for a good long time, or until it stopped working altogether.

Just this hindbrain alone will keep a cold-blooded animal alive. Several bundles or tracts of nerves—those that control the tongue, the throat, the larynx, the digestive tract, the inlets for sound, for the detection of orientation, of balance, are all here. Even the neural sluiceways for tears are discovered here. One can eat, and digest, and cry with nothing more than this. All else above the hindbrain is a refinement of this reptilian brain. In truth, a warm-blooded animal could survive with nothing more than this—if the thermostatic ridges just above were not ravaged. This much could be returned to the world above and, if it were supported by physicians and nurses and machines, live indefinitely.

Cunnought is very still now. He is alert as he moves down, feeling his way, but he is still. Only when his hand reaches up to return an instrument does it quiver. As he moves down, he is still, unhurried, and certain; then again, as the hands rise up, they quiver, are released, and quiver again; first still and sure, then quivering; still and sure, then quivering, fluttering up to gather force again.

The spheres of the cerebellum guide the hands of the painter and of the guitarist and of the surgeon, and guide the canoeist in the continuous infinitesimal adjustments of muscles as he makes his way through the rapids.

When he was a resident, Cunnought saw a young man who had just, some twenty or thirty minutes before, been in an automobile accident. The young man had been arguing with his young wife and had run into a bridge abutment, suffering terrible damage to his face. Cunnought looked into the young man's mouth, and what Cunnought saw made him dizzy. It was, he thought, the most shocking view he had ever had of a cerebellum.

If one would allow an instrument to tap lightly against the brain, a small blush would appear at once—a blush of broken blood vessels, a small blush, almost unnoticeable, that would kill some unfathomable number of neurons. At the Neurological Institute, Dr. Mount would say, hmm, that doesn't look good, does it. Small cotton sponges were placed over the blushing brain.

Now, a neurosurgeon said, narrating a film he had made of one of his operations, this is the point at which I think I might be able to teach you something about proper technique in removing a tumor near the optic nerve. This tumor has pressed against the optic nerve in such a way as to give the patient a right homonymous hemianopsia—blindness, that is, in both eyes, to his right side. The entire field of vision to the right has been obliterated. In removing such a tumor, one must be careful of the approach, for, as you will observe, if your approach takes you too close to the optic nerve, well—(and the movie screen turned completely red).

Here are the ventricles, like the stump and lower branches of a dwarf tree—but hollow, and with the most delicate, onionskin white walls. This place is deep within the center of the brain, and one must proceed cautiously here, for a pinprick hole in these walls will poison the great reservoirs of spinal fluid.

The blood leaks through and is made free of contamination, pure and lucent, filtered by these membrane walls. The filtered blood is the cerebrospinal fluid, and that fluid flows down around the spinal column, nourishing brain and spine. The brain floats in this fluid, is cushioned and protected by it, shielded from the rest of the body by this constant flow of clearest liquid. The brain floats lightly in this tide, suspended in its own cosmos.

Only when this elaborately remote space is invaded can the flow be upset. If the walls of the ventricles become infected, inflamed—if meningitis occurs—or if one of the ventricles becomes pinched off because of an encroaching tumor, the fluid will continue to be flooded into the system, but it will not be reabsorbed, and it will fill the skull with ever-increasing pressure, producing hydrocephalus, pushing the brain out against the skull. Then the walls of the ventricles must be pierced to drain the fluid. If the cisterna magna—the great reservoir at the base of the brain—must be drained, the procedure is performed with great care. A needle must be inserted into the reservoir just so; if the needle pierces the base of the brain, if it penetrates the medulla, the patient dies.

Some things here are known within a micron of precision, within a fiftieth of a micron of exactitude, and much else is darkness, fantasy, monsters, ignorance, brutishness, and sometimes, just along the edge of these two worlds, where the surgeon operates, it is not possible to tell which is which.

The telltale sign is a drop of blood. The needle is placed, and out comes spinal fluid, or a drop of blood. If it is blood, the patient is finished. Cunnought knew of a physician who performed a cisternal tap on a middle-aged woman. He inserted the needle and saw the blood. He stepped around in front to face the patient. Mrs. Edgerton, he said, in a few minutes your worries will be over. And he left the room.

Cunnought had done a tap once and had been greeted with the spurt of blood. He told the nurse just to let him know by way of a signal to his beeper when the man died. Later that day, as he was driving to a Giants' football game with his son, he got the signal.

It no longer occurred to him to invite Janet to go with him to the operating room. He might mention in passing what he had to do one day and he would, from time to time, come back to tell her what he had done, whether it had gone well or badly, what reservoirs and tributaries he had encountered, and she would listen—sometimes enchanted, not always quite comprehending. He had bought two kayaks, but she was not intrigued by the thought of going with him in the rapids. Now his son came along from time to time to practice on the gentler streams. His daughter had come with him once to see him perform an operation on an older woman, who had, unhappily, died in midcourse.

Janet liked to read. She consumed books, inhaled them—and stood back somewhat from the turmoil. Dark-haired, slender, dark-eyed, willowy, warm, somewhat removed.

One Christmas Eve Cunnought had to miss an annual party with family friends in order to perform an emergency operation to remove a tumor near a patient's optic nerve. But, before the patient could be brought to the operating room his heart stopped. The resident phoned Cunnought and said, merely, Merry Christmas. Cunnought's children were delighted to see him home for the party. Hi, Daddy, the patient died?

His father always brought home the unexpurgated stories of the events of the day—psychopathic murderers the therapist had been called in to see, corporate executives with psychosomatic diseases. Cunnought had not been spared these, and even harsher, tales. He had been intrigued by the stories of criminals, whose pictures he had seen in newspapers, by the thought that his father visited them face to face, alone with them in their cells; and his father had taken him to see for himself just how unhappy these dashing criminals were, how unfortunate, how tedious, how lacking in spontaneity, bereft of freedom, for reasons he could not divine, condemned to perform acts that brought them repeatedly back to jail.

Cunnought had started out to be a psychiatrist, but then it seemed to him that he could often intervene earlier and more fundamentally by moving on the structures of the neurons themselves. Much of what occurs in the brain can be explained by electricity and chemistry, by the movement of ions and hormones. Much can be cured or improved by chemistry or by surgery. Much is more precise, more certain, quicker, more decisive, more under one's control in surgery.

When he was a youngster, Cunnought read about a thoracic surgeon who had operated on Arthur Godfrey. After the operation, the surgeon left the hospital and drove down Second Avenue and stopped at a coffee shop for a hamburger. Hey, the counterman shouted, you want catsup on that? The counterman had no idea who the surgeon was, what the surgeon had just done, what secrets he knew, how he had just handled a matter of life and death, how, in fact, he was licensed to deal out life and death, licensed to decide, in a moment, what he must do, whether his act will kill or save a life.

He rode the train from Philadelphia to New York once or twice a year to visit Grandpapa all on his own. Grandpapa would take him into the study to talk about his studies, his days at school, the football team, and medicine, and, as time went on, the ritual would conclude with Grandpapa's gift of a gun from his collection.

Cunnought had once treated a young boy with a malignant tumor. The boy was receiving chemotherapy by way of lumbar spinal injections. In time this approach ceased to work, and

Cunnought switched to injections into the cisterna magna, although it was clear by then that the boy was going to die. After four injections, Cunnought sensed something wrong. He was uncertain what was wrong; he could not account for his unease. He told the boy's doctor that he was afraid that the next time he made an injection he might bump off the boy. Go ahead, the youngster's doctor said, bump him off. The expression in these cases sometimes was: terminate with extreme kindness.

Someone must be prepared to make these decisions, he believed. Most people could not handle such matters. Most people did not want to. Most people wished to leave the decision to another, to be taken care of. Someone had to be able to face death, bear the burden of not knowing, the burden of confusion, and act.

He thought often of the astronaut who was asked what he would do if his last fail-safe system had failed and he had only ten seconds in which to do something. The astronaut said he would think for nine seconds and then act.

Kathy believed in God, he knew; she believed that one is in God's hands upon occasion. He was grateful she had not asked him whether he believed in God.

He would have had to say No. He wondered what she would have said. Really? she would have said.

I hate to say it . . . but I find that the patients I have who believe in God tend to be just not very bright. Or, sometimes, I have to consider whether a belief in God is a symptom of hysteria.

Perhaps that would have been too direct.

Do you think I'm stupid? she would have asked.

No.

Or hysterical?

I think it's almost a prerequisite for anyone who wants to be a performer to be very emotional.

You're just a very cool, rational kind of guy who has all the answers for how things work.

I just have to operate on the assumption that destruction of even a tiny area of the occipital lobe (I don't know just where) of the left hemisphere can cause a permanent blind spot in the right visual field of both your right and left eyes. Destruction of a large portion of the occipital lobe of the left hemisphere can cause complete blindness on the right side. If damage is done to the occipital lobe of the right hemisphere as well, you may not be able to recognize familiar people or places, to tell left from right, to find your way from one room to another, or to picture things any longer in your "mind's eye."

Damage to the parietal lobe can cause a loss of feeling in your right side, loss of the sense of touch, loss of the sense of pain, heat, cold, caress. If you have damage in this area you may not be able to tell whether you have a key in your hand, or a pencil—unless you look. You may not be able to write. You may not be able to strum a guitar. You may not be able to play the piano.

Damage to your temporal lobe may impair your sense of word discrimination; you may not be able to recognize words spoken to you, or find words you wish to use in reply. You may not be able to read, to read newspapers or books or musical notes or to count.

You may read *vase* when you see *antique;* you may read *parrot* when you see *canary*; you may read *pixie* when you see *gnome*. When asked to name a bunch of keys, you may say, as one patient suffering from what is called nominal aphasia said, "Indication of measurement of piece of apparatus or intimating the cost of apparatus in various forms.'' You may have some difficulty with what is called perseveration, as did the patient who insisted upon calling a pair of scissors a nail file until the word *scissors* was finally suggested to him, and he then said. "Yes, that's it! Of course it is not a nail file, it is a nail file.'' You may have both receptive aphasia and expressive aphasia. One patient suffering from word deafness said to his doctor, "Voice comes but no words, I can hear, sounds come, but words don't separate. There is no trouble at all with sound. Sounds come, I can hear, but I cannot understand it.''

One of Wilder Penfield's patients, suffering from syntactical aphasia, described the operation Penfield had performed like this: "Well, I thought thing I am going to the tell is about my operation and it is not about all I can tell is about the preparation the had was always the V time was when they had me to get ready that is they shaved off all my hair was and a few odd parts of pencil they pr quive me in the fanny.''

If you can write at all, you may write like this: "Wlter rolgh was a yound menn m woust to rob sponsch treasure shreps and he was a grote fo fat favout af the Quen and he bunnt the fleat of sbne in the horber and he co cone book and said he had bur the kens of spoin bred.''

If you can speak at all, you may speak like this: "Well now . . . I mean . . . so . . . we . . . now . . . went . . . went . . . suddenly . . . now this . . . like this . . . bang! . . . and then—nothing . . . nothing . . . and since . . . little by little . . . better still . . . quite . . . and now . . . do you see?''

I really hope not, you know.

So do I.

So you know where everything is.

No.

Above the brain stem and the midbrain, the cortex explodes into a vast mushroom cap, divided into two hemispheres and four principal ranges or lobes. At the back of the head are the occipital lobes, those reserved for sight.

Touching—and the other senses of feeling of the body and limbs—is concentrated in the parietal lobes, just in front of the occipital lobes. If a line were drawn from the ear up over the top of the head—and then down the other side to the other ear—just under that line would lie a deep crevice in the cortex of the brain. This fissure, the fissure of Rolando, separates the parietal lobes from the frontal lobes. Just along this fissure, running from just near the ear on up to the top of the head, is a strip of neurons to which all the impulses from the body come. If a fine electrode is placed at the lowest point along this strip, it will produce a tingling sensation in the pharynx and the tongue; somewhat farther up, the electrode will cause a tingling sensation in the teeth, gums, and jaw, and then a very large area is reserved for sensations from the lips. Next comes the sensory area for the face, the nose and eyes—which seem to be not as large, taken all together, as the area for the lips alone. The hands then have one of the largest portions of the sensory strip—as large an area as the whole of the head and lips, larger than the area next reserved for the entire arm and shoulder. A small area is reserved for the neck, a small area for the hips. At the very top of the head is the area reserved for the leg. Then, at the point that the cortex folds down into the deep midline chasm that divides the two hemispheres, a remarkably large portion of the strip is reserved for the foot and toes, and then, far down within the chasm, is a remarkably small area of sensory cortex reserved for the genitals. Interns enjoy speaking of a young woman who had a tumor deep in the midline chasm and so was given to frequent genital seizures. Her husband, it is said, died of a heart attack.

On the other side of the fissure of Rolando, is a strip of motor neurons, that exercise some control over the efferent impulses that go out to the muscles. Beginning again at the bottom of the fissure, the cortical areas are reserved, as in the sensory strip, for tongue, jaw, lips, hand, trunk, and leg. In the motor cortex, areas for control of the mouth—for the areas of speech—seem especially large, as do the areas that control the hands and fingers and, finally, the leg appears to have a greater share of the motor cortex than it does of the sensory cortex.

Where do I sing?

I can't tell you that. I'm not even certain I can tell you where you speak. I can tell you that damage to this area or that may cause difficulty in one part or another of the function of speech—in word recognition, in hearing, in syntactical structures—but I don't know where speech itself resides. Speech requires a sense of discrimination of sounds—and so it requires some help from the temporal lobe. It requires some help from the motor cortex to manipulate tongue and lips. Language use in writing requires help from the visual skills concentrated in the occipital lobes. The simpler actions can be located in a particular place in the nervous system but as the activities become more complex they must draw upon more areas of the nervous system to be carried into effect. Each one of the major lobes of the human cortex appears to have a tremendous area of exclusively associative neurons, neurons that take the impressions transmitted from the senses, from sight and hearing and touch, and from the internal systems of glands and hormones, that draw these impressions together, relate them to one another, compare them to previous similar sensations and determine some suitable response. The more complex a human ability is, the more difficult it is to pin down in any particular area of the brain. Reading and writing and speaking seem to be governed by vaguely defined areas in the left hemisphere—but the expressive use of language is an ability so complex as to be impossible to locate.

At times the patterns coalesce; one region or another of the brain takes on a certain character; one range of hills and valleys seems to form a sound chamber, or a well of speech and a precise and lucid vision forms, like a sudden revelation of bright pebbles beneath the surface of the rapids. Here, it seems, is the center of speech or music, mathematics or logic. And then, just as the shapes have come into focus, they dissolve again and elsewhere, to left or right, another clear pattern presents itself to tempt the gaze, to disappear in splashes of color.

These structures, shapes, imagined patterns—Wernicke's area, Geschwind's syndrome—are as unstable as the pictures of buffalos and dragons to be seen in drifting summer clouds. How much is some reality perceived—how much is a sheer tour de force of imagination—is entirely unknown. There are the blue caverns, violet tunnels, there on the violet hillsides, washed-out banks, violet stands of leafless ash and hemlock, hawthorne and olive intertwined with giant maidenhair ferns, violet streams and boulders. Here we leave civilization far behind, here we lose the fine, precise mechanisms of electrical devices and descend to the realm of chemicals, of acids and of hormones. Here, the pituitary is linked to the brain; it is anatomically part of the brain; it is a nexus of electrical systems and chemical systems and glandular systems. What will you tell me speech is now? Electricity? These neurons?

Here is a oneness of body and brain, from the cells of your toes
to the synapses of your frontal lobes, so hard to fathom that it
would cause pain in the joints of a Christian mystic. Where is
your consciousness now? I think it must suffuse you. Where is
your music now? It must pervade you.

Where is your fear, your anxiety, your rage? In the hypothalamus, here, just next to the pituitary, wells the eight-armed
god of panic and destruction—or here, at least, he appears
from time to time, whether or not this may be his home. Here,
too, the dragon of gluttony may at once materialize. It is not
known whether he lives here, or not; but here he will
appear—so too monsters of fire and thirst. It was here, fifty
years ago, that W. R. Hess, the Zurich mountaineer, placed
fine electrodes in the hypothalamus of a cat, and, when Hess
turned on the current, the cat arched its back, lashed its tail,
snarled, spat, and turned at last—who can be surprised—on
Hess.

Here, sometimes, the form of a fish seems to appear,
smooth and fat, silver-scaled, green-finned, gills of yellow-
green and baby blue, an angry eye, streaked with blood-red
brown, marked with a heavy brow of black, an imperious fish,
haughty, arrogant, demanding, and dissatisfied.

But all these shapes will not so readily form a simile. The
shark with the mouth of blood grows tailfeathers at its nether
end; the paramecium grows the head of a tick, the sail of the
schooner bleeds away into a red and yellow banner, in a ripple,
to an alligator's eye. And then, at last, there is no familiarity in
some of these shapes, for the heavy droplet of deep velvet
green with its black nucleus sprouts a crown of thorns, a flower
pot, a bunch of violets, a hat with soft eyes and flat green nose,
a yellow worm with peacock feathers, apron of baby blue and
crimson, with a blue head (helmeted as a Roman soldier), the

lips of fish with light sun-yellow tubular legs, lampshade chest, the head of a small bird, emerald beak, emerald eyes, ruby crown, tapestried tail and a dog's head with dagger nose, double-chinned and eyeless, lightning bolts, cascades and falls, torrents of consciousness.

This is where the monsters dwell, just down the smooth, spiral path ahead, beyond the dwarf trees on the left, beyond the deep, pink gully, the pink hay-scented ferns, the tendrils of the pruned red laurel, where the path rises to a hillock and then disappears below amid the burnt umber of the hillside, and the pink sky.

I don't see it.

No.

It is here that the throw of a lightning bolt will cause rats, cats, guinea pigs, male and female both, to cease mating. Here, or nearby, fine electrodes will induce erect penises and frequent ejaculation in the male rats and monkeys, prolonged sexual receptiveness in female rats and monkeys. Near this crevice, Peter Milner and James Olds implanted electrodes: the rats who were the subject of their experiment learned that they could turn on the electrical stimulus themselves by pressing levers in their cages; and the rats pressed the lever repeatedly, hundreds of times an hour, without stop, without eating or drinking, until they were too exhausted to continue. They preferred this shocking state of affairs to sex.

Here is the amygdala, named for its resemblance to the shape of an almond. It, too, is deep within the center of the brain. If it is removed, even a wild rat will become tame and quiet. Sometimes. Sometimes, if it is removed, just the opposite phenomenon occurs: the rat becomes more fearful and aggressive. What is this thing? Is this the wellspring of fear? Or is it, perhaps, the source of a sense of territoriality that, if it is damaged, causes an unprovoked attack when we are on our home ground, extreme submissiveness when we are on alien territory? Or is it merely a boulder that, when it is moved aside, releases demons from a cave we had not seen before? Do the demons reside in this place, or merely protect it?

José Delgado placed electrodes in this region of a bull's brain and then the bull and Delgado, equipped with a cape and a radio transmitter, entered a bullring. The bull charged Delgado, and Delgado stopped the animal by sending a message to its amygdala. What monster here has been controlled, or let loose?

What happens when you lose control?

Well, you could die.

You could?

No, *you* could. *You* could die. I'm not speaking in metaphors or hyperboles. You could die.

Is that true?

Of course it is.

Or maybe you'd have to depend on someone else to take care of things.

I'd rather not. I'm an Emersonian. I believe in self-reliance.

More than that, you believe in calling all the shots.

Well, yes.

You tempt the gods to strike you down.

I'll take that risk.

You take it for me, too.

It's too late now to be anything but Prometheus. Neither of us has a choice.

What happened to Prometheus?

Never mind.

Do you think you might ever have suffered from delusions of grandeur?

Never.

Oh, good, then I guess everything's okay.

Perhaps. No one knows just what these frontal lobes are meant to do. They have connecting lines to all parts of the brain, but especially with the hypothalamus and pituitary-gland regions—the regions that control the powerful survival urges—and so they seem to have some special mollifying influence over personality.

In 1848 a young road-worker named Phineas Gage was setting a powder charge, apparently tamping the powder down in a hole with a four-foot iron bar when a spark set off an explosion and the bar was driven neatly up through his left eye and out the top of his head. He was amazed—and stunned for about an hour—but then he got on his feet and walked to see a doctor. "Gage lived for twelve years afterwards," according to a medical journal of the time; "but whereas before the injury he had been a most efficient and capable foreman in charge of laborers, afterwards he was unfit to be given such work. He became fitful and irreverent, indulged at times in the grossest profanity, and showed little respect for his fellow men. He was impatient of restraint or advice, at times obstinate, yet capricious and vacillating. A child in his intellectual capacity and manifestations, he had the animal passions of a strong man." Gage had administered to himself an extemporaneous prefrontal lobotomy.

The prefrontal lobotomy is a simple operation, and, back in the days that doctors made house calls they would often perform a lobotomy right in the patient's home by taking an ice pick (sterilized) and sticking it up through the patient's eye socket, swishing it around a bit, and withdrawing it.

Professor G. Rylander of Stockholm performed a lobotomy on his household cook, and concluded afterward that the qual-

ity of her cooking deteriorated. In an operation that Rylander
performed with Dr. Olof Sjoquist on a woman who was obsessed with the notion that she had sinned against the Holy
Ghost, the surgeons removed a substantial portion of the prefrontal lobe on one side. The operation was done under local
anesthetic, and, having removed this much of the frontal lobe,
the surgeons asked the woman about the Holy Ghost and found
she still believed she had sinned against Him. They cut deeply
into the other side then and asked her again. She was still
obsessed with her sin. They kept cutting, more and more
deeply, until at last she said, ''Oh, I don't believe in the Holy
Ghost any more.'' (The Holy Ghost resides in the fibers of the
medial ventral quadrant.)

You are an atheist, then.

Yes.

And a Republican.

Are these two things related?

You believe that everything is formed by genes, and
neurons, and that nothing can be done to change.

Not nothing.

But little.

Perhaps.

You believe in fate.

Yes.

Not free will.

No.

If you were not an atheist, you would be a Protestant.

I would be a Unitarian.

God help us. What's going to become of me?

What should?

I think in three or four months my hair will have grown back
and I'll be able to sing again.

Most people don't give a damn whether they can sing or not.
Really?

For most people, you know, singing is only a hobby.

Oh, sure. But not for me. Please don't cut out my songs.

Where are your songs? I can't tell you that. Where is your
music?

Memory does not exist in one little track of neurons or
another but as a total impression made up of many bits. We all
have known some memory that seemed to be composed of a
fragment of an image, perhaps a scent, the recollection of a
particular touch, of the feel of a scarf, the sounds of a musical
instrument, or murmuring voices, and of a dozen other bits
that ultimately make up a recollection of a person, of a time, of
a weekend or a moment.

As we age, we appear to lose one bit of information or
another: our neurons commence to die by the time we are
twenty-five years old, and they are not replaced. Bits of
memories may be shunted from place to place in the brain—if,
indeed, they can ever be said to reside in any single place—
but, eventually, the bits may be lost; and then a memory must
be reconstituted from only hundreds rather than thousands of
bits, and then from tens rather than hundreds, so that finally we
may be left with only those memories that are constituted of
the most bits, those that were impressed upon our consciousness in the days that our brain was most actively adding new
impressions at a rapid rate, the memories of childhood. In the
absence of other, clearer recent memories, we recall our child-
hoods over and over again.

Just where these bits, these traces of memory lie, just how
they come to be, how they are maintained, how they are recalled are all unknown. It would be a terrific thing to know
more, because our memories are, in some very essential way,

who we are. Our recollections of our past, of our most important private, secret experiences and of the common things
we have shared with others, with our friends and families,
what we know of the pasts of our fathers and mothers, what we
have taken from the history of the world as our own, what we
recall from myth and literature, from music and painting and
have made our own—all this is who we are and what makes us
each unique. Not even identical twins will finally grow to have
the same memories. They may begin with almost identical sets
of neurons, with certain genetically programmed abilities; but
they will—they cannot prevent it—become unique.

Yet, we cannot find what makes us who we are. Such
miraculous human attributes as a capacity for forethought and
reason, for sympathy, empathy, and love, all of those attributes that make human beings capable of culture, civilization,
and consciousness, all the capacity for wit, humor, in-
ventiveness, novelty, creativity that are, finally, the ultimate
distinctions of the human species, all that makes human beings
human, finally simply disappear within those elusive constellations of the mind.

We should do some opera and some musical comedy and
some Judy Collins.

You'd like to be Judy Collins?

Well, you know, a popular singer. Miss Bampton wants me
to sing opera, and it's true I have a big enough voice, but I
don't think it's what I do best. I like to sing pop songs and
write my own.

Are you good enough to be a star?

I don't know. I think I could have a career. I'm a musician,
you know, star or not. It's my life. I could get along. I've
spent my life at music, you know, no matter how young I am,
it's no joke. It's who I am.

The human brain contains 100 billion neurons—as many neurons as there are stars in the Milky Way—each one of which is divided into a trinity of dendrite (which receives the electrical impulse), the cell body (which contains the nucleus), and the axon (down which the impulse travels to activate a muscle or connect to the dendrite of yet another neuron and send the message traveling onward). At each one of these connection points between axon and dendrite is a space, infinitesimally small, a gap of one fiftieth of a micron—the synapse; the electrical impulse must leap this gap from axon to dendrite in order to carry its message onward; and it is assisted in leaping this gap by small amounts of chemical transmitter substance, neurotransmitters, that carry the tiny explosion across the gap, dazzling the infinitesimal space for an instant of brilliance before the bits of fire fade once more in darkness.

The star will explode or not; it does not linger vaguely in some indeterminate state; it will astonish, or it will not; yet, even so, it is not a simple machine to be turned either on or off; it will explode or not as often as one thousand times a second; it will explode in rhythms; it will erupt in iambs and trochees, in dactyls, spondees, anapests, in ceasura and catalexis. Nor is a neuron an isolated marvel; each cell may have as many as ten thousand synaptic connections with other cells, or even more. Some of the cells of the cerebellum have as many as 300,000 synaptic connections to other neurons. Whether an electrical charge will move along from cell to cell depends not just on one cell relaying its charge to the next. The potential for each single neuron's firing depends upon thousands of explosions from a hundred thousand sources, arriving in a myriad of rhythms, at different rates of speed, detonating just across the space that separates it from the dendrite of the next neuron. Some of these axons that carry the charge are wrapped around the dendrites of the next cell, making thousands of synaptic connections with their neighbors; some axons reach directly to the cell body of the next neuron; some cell bodies are covered with thousands of direct synapses—to be set off, or not, depending upon the sum of all these massive explosions—each one of which depends in its turn upon some one or hundreds of thousands of explosions that occur elsewhere back along the flourishings of synapses of the evanescent spectacle of consciousness.

These neurons are beautiful things—no two of them precisely the same, most of them excessive, sloppy, probabilistic things, delicate versicolored structures, splashes and fierce tendrils of crimson, cadmium yellow, burnt ocher, like the facets of the iris of an eye, and where the web is torn or cut, black to the depths of chaos.

The eye's retina rises from the very center of the brain. When the human embryo has reached the age of seven weeks, two small nubs appear on either side of its midbrain. The midbrain is not otherwise remarkable: it is a focus for several glands, but it is not interesting in any other way but this: the small nubs grow, extend forward, stretch toward the surface of the head and, as they reach the surface, the tips of these shoots form into buds and then open into retinae, into the eyes. The eyes are not merely spheres connected to the brain: they are the brain itself, risen to see the world; and when we look into the eyes of another, we look directly into the brain of another.

The neurons of the brain are not only many millions of beautiful, dazzling, isolated points of energy as the stars of the Milky Way are. The points of energy of the brain are connected to one another in intensely complex, direct, and intimate ways and it is in those connections that our fleeting patterns of awareness and thought exist; it is in these immaterial waves of vanishing connections that our minds are discovered. Nor is each galaxy inside each human skull isolated from others; rather each is connected with billions of others by those unique capacities for language and music, and each is altered and modified by those intangible connections that give rise to a shared sense of identity and reality, of the world and of ourselves.

Nor is each brain merely a summation of present sensations; but rather, because of our capacities for memory—for the passing down of knowledge and culture, of the history and myth that shape the constellations of the human mind, each mind is a mind among minds of present, past, and future; each mind is a mind that is formed and transformed by its awareness of a shared consciousness that exists on a continuum from microcosm to a macrocosm too vast to understand—a macrocosm from which our consciousness seems to spring and to which, in some sense, it returns; a macrocosmic consciousness that would seem to be everywhere and nowhere; a consciousness that is, perhaps omniscient, perhaps omnipotent, that extends backward and forward apparently to infinity, apparently eternally. We can only understand our own minds if we understand them as a part of this transcendent consciousness. And yet, as a matter of simple logic, of elementary reason, our minds cannot comprehend what is greater than the mind itself. We are left with a phenomenon that is inexplicable and that continues to attempt to comprehend itself by efforts of its own imagining, a work of ever-changing science and fiction and theology and poetry.

Three

We seem to be running out of room here, Cunnought said.
Luddy thought he was joking.

I don't think I can see very well. The space here seems to be getting smaller.

Are your glasses okay?

Yes, I don't think there's anything wrong with my glasses.

Cunnought stepped back from the table to look through the magnifying glasses at his own hands. The glasses seemed to be perfectly normal. He looked again at the brain on which he was operating, and it appeared somehow slightly swollen.

How is the anesthetic, Tsing? Everything all right down there?

Everything fine.

Is the patient waking up?

Waking up? No. Certainly not.

Well, what's going on here? I think you'd better check all your lines, Tsing. I think this brain is swelling up. You've given the patient the Mannitol, have you?

Yes.

Cunnought stood back from the table, not moving.

Luddy said he thought the brain looked fine; it looked not at all swollen to him.

No, I think the brain is swelling up. You've checked over everything, have you, Tsing?

Yes.

Everything perfectly normal?

Absolutely fine.

You know people can wake up in the middle of an operation. They feel no pain, but they are awake, and they can't move. It's like being stuck upside down in your sleeping bag. You know that.

Yes, doctor.

Well, this is the damndest thing. Let's do what we can to bring the brain back down. Let's hyperventilate the patient.

Okay.

Let's send off for some blood gases. I think we're in trouble. Let's call in the attending anesthesiologist, just to check us out, right?

Absolutely.

Are you hyperventilating?

Yes. Is the brain shrinking?

No.

Karen, maybe you would see who is available out there, see if there's someone in Room Two who could come and check us out. You know, Tsing, I hope this is your fault. I hope you've done something wrong, because if you haven't, you know, we're in real trouble.

What is it?

I don't know. Have you ever seen anything like this?

No.

We might be having a hemorrhage.

Where?

Somewhere we can't see; there may be a hemorrhage building pressure up against the brain and causing it to rise up toward us.

From where?

Well, from down under somewhere, from the other hemisphere, or perhaps from behind. You know, she's a singer, you know that.

Yes.

This area that is swelling up toward us, this is where she sings, you know, as far as anyone can say, as far as this girl is concerned, this is where she lives.

Yeah.

Jesus, this is awful.

What shall we do?

We'll just stand here for a while, and think about it.

The room was soon flooded with green-clothed nurses and physicians, as Cunnought stood back from the table, his hands held before him, fingers pointed upward, touching nothing. And, as the anesthesiologists read the numbers out to one another—three times around—and felt the tubes for blocks or kinks, opened and closed the intravenous lines, read aloud to one another the entries in the chart, Cunnought gazed across the room at the X-rays and attempted to recall all he had been taught about the blood supply to the brain, all that he had seen in the operating room, all that he had heard of gossip at the conferences, at bedsides, in the doctors' cafeteria.

You know this girl is a singer, did you know that?

What do you have here? You have a deep hemorrhage?

No, not that I can find. No, the brain itself is just swelling and bleeding, all the small vessels there in the temporal lobe are just bursting on their own. What are we missing here, do you see?

No.

Well, let's drain some · spinal fluid—right?—take it right down.

Right.

He stood with hands held immobile, unable to think to do a thing, as her life slipped away from him. Anesthesiologists came and went in the operating room, submerging him in turmoil. They thought that he had made some mistake, but he could not imagine what it could have been, and he stood recalling all that he had done, seeing no misstep.

He could not calculate how much time she had left. Not knowing what was causing this disorder, he could not guess how long he had to act. He must not rush blindly in. He must continue to hold his hands aloft, touching nothing, ready to move should he divine what he had to do. And as he stood and watched, he saw her brain continue to swell; he saw the delicate blood vessels burst and bleed one by one. She had been right, he thought, to have been frightened. She would have said she had been crazy, and he knew she would ask him whether all her shouting and craziness had caused this horror.

No.

Does it happen sometimes?

I've never heard of it. Sometimes, you know, I've heard of patients who were absolutely convinced they were going to die in an operation and then they do. I'm not superstitious, but I try not to operate on someone who's sure they'll die.

It's not a joke.

No, it's not a joke.

Well, if it's too bad, if there's no hope, just make a mistake, just let me go, just let me go, do you understand?

I understand.

He could not conceive what caused this trouble. If he were to try to go down into the center of this explosion, plunging into its midst blindly, thrashing and blundering through the blood, he would only risk some worse disaster, crash into another vein or artery perhaps. He was defeated in this hemisphere. He could do nothing more here but draw back. He might try some astonishing piece of strategy, something completely unprecedented. He might turn the patient over and approach again from the opposite hemisphere. Perhaps the hemorrhage had occurred there, and that was pushing against the brain, causing it to swell up in the left hemisphere. It was an unlikely possibility, but it was the only one Cunnought could imagine he had left. To turn the patient over, to cut again through flesh and skull, to expose the brain on that side too, was a desperate maneuver. Cunnought could not recall whether any of the four hundred ancient trephined skulls at Harvard showed any evidence of such ruthless practice. The brutality of the maneuver might kill her. The breaking of the sterile operating field that would occur when she was turned would bring the risk of fatal brain infection to the very edge of certainty. Yet, she had no other chance.

Okay, let's turn the patient over and shave the right side, he said to Luddy, and put in a burr hole to see if we find any bleeding there, because I think that is the only strategy we have left. Otherwise I think she is absolutely dead. Any other ideas? Okay, do you want to get ready to turn the patient, Tsing? Cunnought began at once to reach under the sterile cloths that protected the field of operation from infection. He turned the entire field upside down, and Anne was stunned to see him break the field in this way; Luddy suddenly thought that Cunnought had made an insane mistake. Karen thought the patient must already have died. None had ever before seen the field broken in this way.

Cunnought turned the head swiftly and reached without looking for the straight razor that was handed him. He shaved the scalp with a half-dozen uncannily quick strokes of the razor, splashed the skull with disinfectant, seized the knife and cut to the bone in one motion, laid back the flap, leaving control of the superficial bleeding to Luddy. He slipped off his top layer of gloves, retaining the second pair he always wore in a gesture to the sanctity of the sterile field, took hold of the air drill, and burrowed into the skull. Bone curled up the drill bit, and Cunnought prayed he would soon strike blood.

When you're dealing with something like this, you really can't try to second-guess yourself. What really pisses me off are these Monday-morning quarterbacks. Only one person can make the decision, finally. I can't take a poll. I can't wake the patient up and say, hey, what do you think, shall we go ahead and do it? I feel much better when I'm absolutely in control. As far as that goes, when I present the initial proposition to a patient about whether or not to have the operation itself, I can structure the situation to get the answer that I think is best. With an operation for a disk, or some other piece of optional surgery, it's different. Then I present all the information, and the patient decides. But in the case of a tumor, I know the patient must be operated on, and I relieve the patient of the burden of the decision. Most people aren't capable of making life-and-death decisions about their own lives. They don't have the experience or the strength. They find a doctor they can trust, and they go with him. They have to. When you fly in an airplane, you don't ask the pilot a lot of questions. You trust him, or you go elsewhere. I structure the situation so that the patient decides to do what I want the patient to do. I say, here is the way it is; this is what we are prepared to do; this is what I would do—and the patient is usually so relieved to be given a way out of a bad situation that he says, okay, doc, you just do what you think best.

If a patient asks a lot of questions, he is in trouble. When I was a resident, a Good Humor salesman was always asking the doctors and nurses why this and why that and cried wolf all the time and irritated the nurses so that one time when he was sitting on the floor—and he was too weak to get up—the nurses just left him there for four hours, and he got cold, caught pneumonia, and died. He just died of obnoxiousness.

Well, you can't second-guess these things, that's all. It just makes me goddam mad when you've done the best anyone could have done—you've had all the knowledge and all the skill, and if you look at it without sentimentality and just be a little cold and hard-headed about it, the absolute fact of the matter, and you know it, is that you have absolutely, unequivocably done the unequivocal right and best thing that could be done, it just pisses me off to be second-guessed.

He was going down near the right temporal lobe now, and no one knows what this area of the brain quite does. Cunnought knows only this: if he plunges the drill down into the brain and causes damage, she may not be able to discriminate among musical notes any longer, or among complex rhythmical combinations; she may no longer recognize music, or be able to sing.

Going down the Allagash, Cunnought says, if you are really good you don't like to take risks. You like to do something amazing that no one else can do, but if you take a foolish risk and luck out, you don't feel good, you just feel stupid. You have to follow the rules; but what really enrages you is if you've followed all the rules and then something goes wrong, and you've lost control, and then you're trapped, being carried along by the rapids and you can't get it right, and that's when you find out you're suddenly all alone and the patient is dying, and you can't turn back, and that's when you have to work against the panic, and that's when you're saying to yourself that ordinarily the worst cases that come in are people who have fallen or been shot in the head, and if they are bleeding to death you can always say to yourself as this guy at Roosevelt said one night, ''Boy, whoever shot this bastard sure killed him''; and then you're just dealing with what you've got and trying to make the best of it, but, when you contract to bring someone into the operating room who is just in need of an operation, just in need of having a tumor removed, say, then you have a contract with yourself, a private contract that you let with yourself that you are going to do better than you usually do, and this person is going to come out better, not like this, not hemorrhaging, not bleeding to death.

Cunnought lifted the drill and let it bounce on the table as he reached for the knife again and flicked open the dura. He put a clip on the dura, flicked again, and looked down into the right hemisphere of the brain. He saw no blood. There was no hemorrhage.

Oh, goddammit, there's no bleeding here, dammit. There's no way to control that swelling. Goddammit. Wouldn't you think draining the goddam spinal fluid would help?

You'd think so.

Son of a bitch. That's it. That's all. That does it. Let's just close up this side and turn the patient back again. Just close it up; I don't think you need to try for a nice cosmetic closing. Not too many people will have a chance to see what kind of stitch you've used on this head.

Cunnought turned from the table and took several steps back

toward the corner, where he stood considering previous operations, Cushing's texts, the operating room monologues of
Pool and Mount, anecdotes, jokes—anything that might be
related to sudden swelling of the brain in the midst of an
operation.

I'll have another pair of seven and a halfs and one of eights,
he said quietly, and he put them on with great deliberation.

We'll take off another piece of bone now from the left
hemisphere and give the brain room to swell without cutting
itself up on the edge of the opening. I'll take the electric saw
again, please. And he carved another hunk of bone out of the
skull, and threw it on the floor. We are now using, he said, the
latest surgical techniques of the eighth century. B.C.

He had given up all hope now. He had cut away a piece of
bone, to give the brain more room to swell, only because it
was his habit not to quit. He would give the brain room to
explode, and hope it might soon subside of its own accord or
that, in another few minutes, he would think of some other
unheard-of strategy. Yet, as he looked at the brain, and saw
the bleeding, distended mass begin to turn the disgusting dull
yellow color of death, he understood that he continued to hack
at the skull in this way, with the outlandish wish to save some
few neurons from being squeezed to death, only because it was
his habit to continue to operate beyond all hope.

He walked around Anne's instrument table and over to the
windows looking out on the Cathedral. Up close to the
windows, Cunnought had a fine view of the north end of
Central Park, nicely blanketed with snow and, from this dis-
tance, seemingly clean. He wished it would snow. He loved to
look up from the operating table and see snow falling in front
of the Cathedral. He considered the X-rays taped to the
window. Beginning with the hindbrain, he considered various

dysfunctions of the autonomic nervous system, of breathing and heartbeat, of rapid alterations in cerebrospinal fluid, chemically induced spasms, various forms of seizures, fits, the effect of curare, sublimaze, sodium pentathol, and nitrous oxide on the central nervous system, of cataclysmic allergic reactions, of the blood supply system, tracing the carotid artery through its principal branches, moving carefully up into the temporal lobe, retracing the pathways, back down and up again another route, back down all the way to the basilar artery, and similarly up along its branches and rivulets. He was lost, in this way, for some five or ten minutes, reviewing, as best he could, all he knew that might in some way bear upon the disaster of this inexplicable rising up, as though of some primitive monster, to savage this life, to lay it waste even in the very presence of all of the most sophisticated knowledge and technology of medicine, even in the very sanctum of the operating room where the control of the physician was at its most powerful and complete.

If the patient's heart or respiration had failed, Cunnought would have understood and known what must be tried. But this swelling of the brain was entirely without precedent in his experience, without precedent in the books he knew, in Cushing or Horrax or even in those light, speculative books by Steven Rose or Luria. It had not been mentioned by Horowitz and Rizzoli, nor presented as a case study at the society of neurosurgeons.

We can find no explanation, doctor.

Cunnought looked back into the operating room. It was now filled with anesthesiologists and nurses, interns and residents, attendings, a radiologist, and all were silent. Cunnought returned to the head of the table.

I know.

The left temporal lobe had swelled angrily and come up and out through the opening of the skull; brain had pushed out and ravaged itself against the edges of the opening in the skull. The brain had stopped beating; it was puffed up and bloody, yellow and ugly. Some of the veins on the surface of the cortex had turned black: here, no blood flowed; it was stagnant.

A voice came over the intercom: Dr. Cunnought?

What?

Dr. Pratt wants to know how everything's going.

What?

Dr. Pratt wants to know how everything's going today, with your operation.

(A silence.)

You can tell Dr. Pratt that she's dead.

What was that?

She's dead! You heard me, goddammit!

Cunnought released the tenting sutures that held the dura away from the opening in the skull and tried to pull the two sides of the thin covering back together to stitch it closed. But the brain protruded too much: and the dura would not stretch to close over the swollen brain.

It was not possible at all to put the bone flap back on the skull. The brain would not be protected either by dura or bone.

Jesus, this is awful.

Cunnought left the brain exposed and went ahead to remove the clamps from the laid-back flap of scalp, to close the muscle tissue and scalp over the naked brain.

God.

He pulled the flap of skin and muscle over the open skull, but it would not stretch to cover the distended brain.

Oh, Jesus. I can't even close.

Brain, smashed against the rough opening of the skull,

raked against the ragged periphery of bone, torn and crushed
and bloody, disgorged itself from the skull.

Oh, God.

You think you could figure out how to close this, Luddy?

The brain is too swollen. There's no room to close.

Oh, isn't there?

Cunnought suddenly plunged his forefinger and middle
finger down into the mutilated brain and scooped out enough
bloody brain to fill a small child's hand, and he turned and
spun—

Oh, shit!

—and threw the clot of brain across the room, against the
wall, spattering antiseptic green walls with blood and brain.

No one in the operating room moved or spoke. Anne felt
light-headed, as though she might faint, and she gripped the
edges of the instrument table and tried to bow her head to let
the blood flow back. Luddy hoped that if he didn't breathe,
Cunnought would not speak to him. The others in the room
stared at the surgeon, unable to look away. And Cunnought
looked at his hands for some few minutes.

He hoped that she was dead, for the brain that stuck to his
fingers was yellow, horrid stuff, and much of the brain that
remained in her skull was worthless stuff, and without attempting to remove the brain that adhered to his hands, he looked up
at the others at last and said, There. Now there's room to
close. We'll prepare the body for autopsy.

He stepped back up to his table, and reached up without
looking, took a suture from Anne, and placed it firmly through
Kathy's scalp, and on down through the mutilated brain,
sewing scalp and brain together. He took another suture and
stitched again through scalp and brain—making Luddy now
feel dizzy—and he continued in this way, one suture after

another, pulling the bloody head back together, when his friend Mimi came into the operating room, and, sensing at once that everyone was stunned and appalled, asked him what had happened, and he replied that he had killed her—no, the others said—and he said nothing more and finished up and peeled off his gloves and dropped them on the floor. When at last the drapes were all removed, and she lay again naked on the table, her head now wrapped prettily in a white turban dressing, he moved around the operating table to her side and, hesitating momentarily, he reached over to touch her eyelid and to look a while into her eyes. Her pupils were fixed and dilated. She might linger for a day—or two at the most.

He turned and left the operating room then. He avoided looking at the others in the room or any of those, nurses and doctors, whom he passed in the corridor on his way to the doctors' locker room—except for Dr. Palamara, who was in charge of the recovery room just then and stopped Cunnought in the hall to ask whether there were anything in particular he might do for this new patient on her way from the operating room, to whom Cunnought said no, don't do anything heroic, it's better if she dies, no, even if she lives she'll only be a gork, just don't do anything heroic—and, in the doctors' locker room he went at once to the telephone and sat down to speak to Patrick.

Patrick had gotten up late that morning and turned on the television set for company and taken his time getting dressed and having a cup of coffee, because he had had nothing to do but wait for the doctor's phone call at four o'clock in the afternoon. Patrick, the doctor said, and Patrick knew at once that the operation had gone wrong, I've got some very bad news for you. Kathy's brain swelled during surgery.

Is she alive?

Yes.

But what?

She's going to die within a day or two.

The doctor was standing out on the pavement on the side of the hospital near the Cathedral, still in his green operating clothes, when Patrick arrived to ask if there were any chance at all, and Cunnought answered no. Was she in any pain? No, none. Did she know what was going on? No, certainly not. You know, Patrick told the doctor, Kathy and I were a team, and there's no such thing as one person on a team.

They went up together to the recovery room, and Patrick saw her—her head was wrapped in neat, pristine white bandages; and it looked quite safe and soft and well-protected and perfectly under control, although it occurred to Patrick that it seemed as though she might have had her whole brain removed, she seemed so peaceful; and she was surrounded by machines and monitors with flashing lights, intravenous tubes and the large tube that went right down her throat, and he took Kathy's hand and prayed.

Why did it happen, Cunnought did not know, never had he seen such a thing before, everything was checked and double-checked, and no one could explain it, these things just happen sometimes, once in a million, or in a billion, or something never seen before, and no one can explain it, is she going to die?

Yes, she is. I'm sorry.

Downstairs again he phoned his uncle Jeremy. Well, I'll be right there. You know, Patrick, I always thought Kathy was the one in our family who was going to achieve something, but now it's up to you, Pat.

And he called Chris who called Eileen who called Liz who fell down on the stove. Jay came to visit at the hospital knowing nothing and heard the doctor give her forty-eight hours to live and Jay then, it seemed to Patrick, went into a glass bottle. Father Wurlin stood in the main entrance of the hospital crying. Chris was white, one arm around Patrick. We have to control ourselves, said Eileen, for Patrick's sake. If a person is cremated, does she still get to have a proper funeral? Someone hit the wall—not anyone that Patrick remembered knowing, the relative, perhaps, of some other patient. Does anyone have a match? Chris cried and left to take a walk. Father Wurlin mentioned the Book of Job.

You realize, the social worker said to Patrick, that if she had lived she would be completely paralyzed. Would you rather have her live like that or rather have her die?

I guess I'd rather have her die.

Well, that proves you love your sister.

When Jay was ten years old, the cops came to the door and told him his father had been killed in an automobile accident.

She was supposed to sing at my wedding, you know.

We're all the same, she said, we all came in at the same time, we have to go out at the same time.

What happened, Patrick?

Rob and Shirley had been drinking and wanted some black coffee.

Hey, what are you doing? Because if you're not doing anything you could come over to the hospital.

Oh, yeah, how come?

Because Kathy Morris is here, you know, and she's dying.

My father works at a hospital in Jersey, and he got this neurosurgeon to call Cunnought, and he says she hasn't got a chance.

Alvin was stoned.

You know, no matter what they say, there's always a chance.

Yeah.

I was listening to "Kind of Blue" by Miles Davis, you know what I mean, which is very cool, very bluesy, you know, very laid back.

My father told me he had a dream years ago that he and I had been in a car wreck, and I was in a hospital crying and saying why, over and over again, why, why, why.

Everyone knows I'm emotional, so I didn't feel very welcome, I thought I ought to stay away, but I couldn't do that, so I'm just trying not to say anything, not even get near to Patrick, because eleven years ago when Mary Beth's father died, Debbie said, the last thing Mary Beth needs is you going, Oh, your father died, oh my God, so that's why I'm just sitting here, and not saying anything.

When I was driving up, Patrick, I was trying to think of some advice to give you. While I was driving, I was thinking what to say, and I couldn't think of any advice to give you.

Patrick went upstairs. He had Cunnought's sports jacket around his shoulders, and the nurses on the floor gave him some pillows and a blanket to take with him into the room where the patients sometimes gathered to watch television or read or play cards, and he found a chair there and thought how he had always said, whatever happened, he could always take one more thing, that always just one more thing could be borne somehow, but he decided not to say that again, because he believed that if he were to say one more thing, then it would be sure to happen. So, no, he could not bear one more thing.

Cunnought had changed by now and could not remember what he had done with his jacket, but he had got back into his white coat, because he must, he knew, pay one last visit to the recovery room before he left the hospital, but he would make his rounds first among the living, although, as he did so, he could not quite see the patients because of the image that stayed before him of the brain that was spattered on the green-tiled wall.

He was, he supposed, thankful that she was dead, or would be soon, since he could not bear to conceive how cursed she would have been to survive half-blind, half-paralyzed, half-deaf, and speechless, condemned to bed, to living death. Yet—who knows?—he would himself wish to live even if he were half-blind, even if he were half-deaf. He would not care to live if he could no longer operate, if he had to give up his surgery, his chance to lose himself several times a week amidst the terrors of his explorations. He could not give up who he was, any more than she could bear to live without her music, but if he were paralyzed, he thought, he could learn to operate with his left hand alone. He could visualize all he needed to know without being able to speak. He could perform his surgery somehow, he thought—or perhaps not. No doubt, in any case, because of what he had seen of the horrible destruction of her brain, she was, no doubt, better dead.

In the recovery room, whose walls, too, are of the same light green that pervades the operating room, Cunnought stood for some time looking at the seemingly sleeping girl, seemingly peaceful and content despite even the tubes and intravenous lines and electrical monitors. He thought that she was a wild, and sometimes violent, passionate girl, and he wished again, that he could hear her sing and know that he had given voice to her song, or wished that he could hear her rage.

Yet, all this was sentimental stuff, for she was better dead and, as for him, he had less and less tolerance for these soft sentiments as time went on; his skill was what was wanted, not his ardor; he had to discover some way to perform his surgery with simple competence and not make it somehow into some extraordinary form or act of love. That was all, he was done, there was nothing more that he could do but let her go.

And so he turned to drive back home, and turned again to look at her. At last, unable finally to turn away without touching her again, he reached out gently with his fingers and opened one of her eyes, and then at once he was stunned and terrified, for her pupils were no longer fixed and dilated; they reacted to the light; they moved.

PART THREE

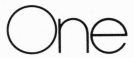

One

11 P.M. B/P stable. NSR—sinus tach. MAI 40%—assisting—Head dressing dry and intact. Moving L. extremities. Opening eyes, but not in response to verbal stimuli. Clear amber urine.

Patrick now stood next to Cunnought, watching. He wondered whether she could feel anything and was assured that she could not. He was pleased that he would have a sister, but he wondered whether or not she would be a vegetable.

11:50 P.M. Pupils slightly unequal. Right pupil slightly larger. B/P 104/70. Does not respond to verbal stimuli. Moves arm and leg on L. side, no movements on R. side.

Patrick thought perhaps that they had not been good enough Christians. He wondered what God meant by it; he wondered what attitude or series of acts or appearance of behavior he might adopt in order to produce some effect on the outcome.

1:15 A.M. Patient taken off respirator. Patient sometimes responds to verbal stimuli. Responds to command squeeze

> hand with L. hand. Cannot move R. side. Responds to com-
> mand breathe deeply. Moves L. leg at intervals. Sometimes
> does not respond to verbal stimuli.

Something was going to survive, and Cunnought was overcome by a sudden flood of memories of the breaking of sterile
procedure in the operating room, and with a sudden dread of a
brain infection that would kill what attempted to survive. He
ordered the nurses to administer a full range of antibiotics and
to wake her up from time to time, rouse her up to consciousness, no matter what the nurses had to do, to pinch her arm or
shoulder or, if that did not make her squirm and groan, to grind
their knuckles in the center of her chest—and, if that failed to
provoke a response, grinding hard, and harder—to call him at
once.

> 9:08 A.M. Patient has made no attempts to talk. Responds to
> painful stimuli. Sometimes responds to verbal stimuli. L.
> hand grip sometimes strong. No movements elicited from R.
> extremities.

She thought that the nurses were very fat with white faces
and peaked caps and painted lips, like the clowns' faces on the
walls, which were sometimes dim and indistinct, as though a
child had drawn them there with crayons, and the skull that
peeped out from behind the arras had painted lips, too, and
blue eye sockets, dark-blue nostrils with a bow tie. The music
teacher had his fingers in his ears, and he frowned; his nose
was red, and tears streamed from his eyes. The conductor's
baton was broken at the end; a fly perched on the end of his
nose, and the first violinist had an upturned cornucopia on his
head. The singer stuck out her tongue, and tears and flies came
out, and she sang Ho Yo Ho To Yo, and the dead cat, splayed
and wild-eyed, fell down from the ceiling.

The judge, or music critic, had a hole in his head just to the left of the center of his forehead. He pointed to it absently and could not help smiling. Two other critics, one on each side, laughed uproariously, without making any sound, and a leg was on the table before them, having been cut off just below the knee. The bloody knife lay on the table next to the leg, and the handsaw with it, along with dentures, a nose, and pen and ink. A man held his head and cried; flies came out of his mouth.

One clown was naked and emaciated, with unruly red hair and large ears, bat ears, ears that grew to the size of elephant's ears and turned white and then yellow and black, to match the striped yellow and black bat wings and six pairs of eyes in the middle of his forehead, hands with feathered flames, the flesh showing through his face, as though the skin had been flayed to reveal the bleeding understructure.

The teacher leered and sang, and his blue eyes liquefied, ran down his face, and his flesh melted to skeletons in the sky filled with scythes, and a flying, toothless candle, a dead, spotted, leering skull with smoking candle eyes and deliquescent teeth, liquid white bone as soft as a percale sheet, bloody red and white, and bright eyes within the skull and flies within and without and flies upon the sheet, flies within the mouth, and flies on arms and legs, flies within the hair and the dustmop, flies within the beard of Christ, the eyes of Christ, the crown of thorns, the open wound, flies within the mouths of mothers, flies within the clothes and beds and coffins of mothers—the conductor laughed, and the soprano sang, her teeth fell out of her mouth and down upon the book of music that she held, notes upon the body of her mother, notes crawling upon the flesh of her dying mother, notes flying up from the dying flesh of mothers, music from the death of mothers, notes of mothers, crawling notes of children, notes of divas, notes of fat ladies of girls in dresses, notes of cakes and cookies, notes of flowers of ducks of sparrows of canaries, notes of butterflies notes of lemons and of wicker baskets, notes of daffodils, notes of maidenhair ferns, notes of celery, notes of apples, notes of sunlight, notes of pastel blue, notes of hillsides of grass, notes of woodlands, notes of forest, notes of ocean sunset, turquoise notes of evening, notes of birdsong of blue crystal, of cello and of flageolet, notes of trumpet, bugle, trombone, notes of drum, of cymbal, bass drum, snare, whistles of the parade of marching, notes of feet of cheers of laughter.

She's dead, someone whispered, she's dead.

It seemed to her not quite like hell, not at all like heaven; she could not understand what the nurses were doing there, nor why the man who stood among them had flowers in his hair, and painted red lips, mascara marks upon his dimples, one on the left side, one right, mascara on his eyes, and a weak chin it was, and a white lace ruff around his neck, and they all stared at him with painted wooden eyes, smiling with wooden teeth, and faces painted white and deep blood red, snarling with still-wet lipstick, moist and glistening, while, once in a while, suddenly the wooden eyes would come alive and shift from side to side and then go dead again.

As the parade went by, she picked out the people she knew: the skeleton in the red skirt and flowered hat, the horse with the bloody dagger, the old man with the white hair and long, thin nose, the bald man with the false rubber nose, the bun-faced man with two bright green eyes set closely together, and the old lady with the white dress and fool's cap, the head that walked alone on dog's feet and wore a monocle, and the elephant that ate the tuba player head first. All these, by now, she knew quite well.

Hurry up, she said. Hurry up.

No one replied; she realized that she might not be speaking out loud.

Hurry up, she said.

Patrick was startled. He thought she had spoken.

What?

Hurry up.

What?

Hurry up!

He could not make out the words, but he began to shout and run for the nurses, asking for the doctor, saying that she had made a sound, running to the corridor, asking for the nurses, calling for the doctor, returning to her bedside.

Hurry up.

The nurse called for the doctor, and wrote in Kathy's chart: Patient can say "It hurts."

Cunnought came and stood by her bed for several minutes. She reached out and took his hand. Hurry up, she said.

Two

Patrick wandered the corridors, saying to the woman in the cafeteria that his sister was alive, that she had spoken and that she was going to live, saying good morning to the guards who roamed the halls, stopping to look at the woman mopping the floor, passing on to the front door and going out for a stroll around the Cathedral. He saw Chris and Liz and Mark out on the street and told them the news, and they all laughed, and Patrick brought them back inside the hospital and up to the room where Kathy lay.

Kathy did not speak, but she did reach out to take Chris's hand and kiss it, and then she said:

How much?

What?

How much?

How much what?

How much?

Do you mean how long?

How much?

Did you say shut up?
How much?
Help me?
How much?
How much what?
How much?

And so Patrick explained how much she had been through, how she had been through an operation, when the operation had occurred, what had happened in the operating room, how everyone had thought that she was dead, how they had seen now that she was alive, how everything would now be fine.

It seemed to Patrick that she improved hour by hour, rapidly. She went back and forth, in and out of consciousness—speaking, then silent, aware, then hazy, lucid, then vague—but, still, hour by hour she was coming back to life bit by bit.

Both Jay and Alvin were allowed to visit her in the Intensive Care Unit, although Jay visited only occasionally and, when he did, he merely stood silently, resting his hand on hers. Alvin visited every day, sometimes twice a day, and he spoke to her, believing that a stream of conversation about normal, everyday things would bring her back to normal, everyday consciousness; and so he told her what he had done that day, whom he had seen, about the need to take his saxophone to the repair shop to have a couple of pads replaced, and how a spring seemed to stick when he played open G, of how he was trying to get up a gig with Harold and Eddie but that Eddie had had to hock his electric piano and Harold had been busted for possession so that Alvin had had to look for some other guys and he had spent the past couple of days trying to frame a note to put up on the school bulletin board that would contain just the right sense of seriousness and humor, the need for classical training but a wish and flair for experimentation with new forms, when he had run into Rob, also putting up a note, hadn't seen him since no one could remember when so they went off together to see *One Flew over the Cuckoo's Nest* with Jack Nicholson about this guy in the hospital who has a lobotomy and never makes trouble again but is going to be peaceful and calm and not run away but stay around where everyone knows where he is from now on and people can take care of him and he won't shout at them or put them down or have them on any more but, in fact, probably be a lot happier than he ever was before although like Rob was saying the Indian certainly had a point, if Rob understood it, about how the Indians had been deprived of their territory and probably should be given large reservations at least to live on although they certainly shouldn't think they had any right any more to lands that had oil on them, because, after all, they might as well be realistic.

She closed her eyes very slowly and banged her fist upon the bed and shook her head.

Hurry up.

How much what?

Hurry up.

And so he explained once again what she had been through, how the disaster had occurred in the operating room, how everyone had thought that she was dead, how everything would now be fine.

She shook her head and smiled and stuck out her tongue and shook her head.

Hurry up.

Patrick looked around the room for help, but neither Chris nor Liz nor Mark could understand what she had said.

Ready. Hurry up.

It's finished, Patrick said. The operation is over.

Uncle Jeremy arrived wearing a cranberry-colored sweater and went directly to Kathy's bedside. She opened her eyes. She said nothing. But, for a moment she appeared to see him; then tears came to her eyes. Jeremy reached down and touched her cheek lightly, stroked her cheek, and said very quietly into her ear, I love you, over and again, shh, I love you, and he left smiling reassuringly—but then he cried, for the first time that he could remember since before his mother had died.

Abigail helped him from the room.

She could hear Patrick speaking to her, but he was far away, at the far end of the white-tiled, antiseptic tunnel, dizzy at the edges, and she was afraid that they had come to hurt her again, so she pretended that she wasn't there. She closed her eyes and pretended she was gone. They talked about her, that she knew; they stood around her and talked about how she was dead. She felt no pain, or perhaps she did; perhaps what she felt was pain, but she could not be certain that this feeling was what was called pain. No, she felt perfectly fine. She could talk and run and jump; she could play ball and sing; she could have a cup of coffee and take a walk down Broadway, all these things she could do even though she was dead.

The doctor with the flowers in his hair came by to hurt her every now and then, and she could not understand how they had let him in to do these things. How much? she asked.

Occasionally, when she had a lucid moment, she realized that she was a vegetable.

Then the intern came who had eyes all over his face, hollow eyeballs like pitted olives connected to one another with long white tendons intermixed with feathers and pieces of raw fish, nostrils and, inside his dry mouth, a baby chicken.

She stuck out her tongue.

How much?

She shook her head.

She banged her fist.

Hurry up.

She smiled.

Hello.

She stuck out her tongue.

She wished that they had not tied her down in bed. She could not move if they kept her tied down this way. She could not bend her knee or bend her arm. She wished that she could turn over on her side and curl up, but she could not move when they had her tied down this way. She wished that she could turn on her other side. She clenched her fist and closed her eyes.

She wished that they would not tie her hands this way. The silk scarf that someone put over her bandage to make her look pretty kept falling down over her eyes, and she could not push it up again. She shook her head from side to side, but she could not move the scarf; it eased down even more over her eyes, and she thought that she might cry.

She wished that someone would turn off the television set. She did not want to watch *The Wizard of Oz*; it made her sick and dizzy. She thought of the stuffings in the scarecrow; she thought the tin man was filled with sawdust; she hoped the tin man would not be taken apart. Every time someone turned on the television set, the same movie was being shown, and it made her feel light-headed. She closed her eyes and pretended that she was not there.

She wished the nurses would not make her sit up in a chair. Her head hurt, and the scarf slipped over her eyes, and she thought that she was slipping sideways and sliding out of the chair onto the floor. She couldn't stop herself; she felt that she was falling; she couldn't speak; she wished they wouldn't put her in the chair and forget about her there. She thought that if she would kick and kick, then at least they would keep her tied down in her bed and not sit her up in the chair again, and so, when she got back into the bed, she kicked and kicked.

She wished they would not bring her food and tie her arms so that she could not eat.

She wished she could tell whether her brother was really there with her or whether she only imagined he was there.

She wished they would untie her hands so she could masturbate, to see if she were dead.

She wished they understood that they had made a mistake, that they had the wrong person, that they were doing the wrong thing to the wrong person.

She wished they would not keep her in chains.

She wished that person would not keep saying, "I think I saw her eyes move."

> Patient awake and responsive to verbal stimuli. Moving all four extremities but does not move right arm very frequently or upon command. Recognizes visitors when they speak to her. Has difficulty speaking but occasionally makes appropriate verbal response. Seems to be aware when she makes appropriate verbal response and becomes frustrated when unable to make appropriate response.

She was moved from the Intensive Care Unit back to an ordinary room.

Sometimes she smiled. Sometimes she would shake her head from side to side. Sometimes she would close her eyes and bang her fist down on the bed. Sometimes she would say Hello.

All this lasted for several days.

Patient not moving right leg or arm at all this evening.
Dressing on head dry and intact.
When awake becomes very agitated and thrashes about in bed.
Speaks incoherently. When calmed down seems to understand what is said to her, and is able to make some coherent statements.
Patient needs to be reassured very often.
Patient becomes calmer when reassured.
Patient alert and restless at times.
Attempts to speak and appears to make sense when able to talk.
Awake—responds readily to verbal stimuli.

All this lasted for several days. Alvin visited each day.

Patrick slept late, and when he remembered his dreams, he remembered his dream that Kathy had one eye, blackened, and that she stared at him without speaking. In the mornings, he drank coffee and watched television and sometimes went back to bed for a nap before lunch. Sometimes he slept until the middle of the afternoon, and then he watched television again until it was time to visit Kathy. He let his car acquire parking tickets—a ticket a day for fifty days, more or less. He had taken two days to drive to Delaware to withdraw from school and pack his things. He wondered whose fault it had been, and he reckoned that he would never know and that there was nothing that he could do, even now that he was the man of the family.

Pupils reactive to light.
Patient alternates periods of self-initiating verbalization with periods of lethargy.
Patient able to follow simple commands.
Remains lethargic but less so than yesterday. Only time patient seems oriented is when she is placed in a chair. At

these times she said "Down me" repeatedly. Becomes extremely restless and agitated and appears uncomfortable. Patient states "It hurts."

Pupils briskly reactive to light. Patient able to verbalize "Hurry up," "Yeah," "Fine," "I don't know."

All this lasted for several days. Alvin visited every day.

A young nurse, Nina, loosened the bonds that held her. Arm restraint loosened, Nina wrote in the chart, and patient thankful. Eyes brightened. Patient is constantly banging left arm against bed in annoyance. Is alert and obeys commands only when she wishes to be cooperative. Patient bangs foot autistically against bottom of bed. I allowed patient to bite finger earlier in day when administering medication and in afternoon, when arm restraints were removed, I allowed patient to hit me for about ten minutes. After episode of hitting, patient held hand and stared, wanting to be calm, wanting to touch me. After this patient in room alone, blurted out several sentences. Only oh God, oh God could be discerned. Remainder inaudible.

Jay came often to the hospital and stayed on the edges, letting Alvin and Patrick stand closest to the bed, feeling he no longer had a claim on Kathy, and at night, he went to Stryker's and played the drums. He dated no one else. He withdrew from school. He thought of going on the road.

She wished she would not keep seeing the flies crawling on the ceiling or the conductor with the broken baton or any more of the clowns or loud trumpet players or the music critic with the flies coming out of the hole in his head, the doctor with the flowers in his hair and nose who kept pressing his fist and knuckles into her chest and along her sore ribs until she could not help but shudder.

But, then, the notes of blue teachers and broken batons conducting blood, conducting trumpets, conducting parades of notes of mothers, notes of yellow birds, wailing fathers, oh, say goodbye to your mother, Patrick, notes of unborn infants, notes of flies upon the tongues of children and their mothers, notes of mothers fallen on the floor, notes of mothers rising from the still body lying on the floor, oh God.

For, there, a woman lay, wide-eyed, with painted red lips, broad hips, a second set of smiling teeth just on her collar bone, a purple breast, blood red stomach, yellow shirt, high-heeled patent leather shoes with black thongs around the ankles—this was not her mother come to get her—taking a white shirt, a man's shirt, or a white nurse's dress off her shoulders, falling to the side, over and over, tumbling into flesh-colored cigarette ashes, a patch of green grass, marble gravestone: she looked down upon herself, laughing uncontrollably, hideously, bright-eyed, laughing, and falling backward, down through the gaping rip in the sheet, down, down through the splashing white, lightning flashes, cataracts of baby blue flame, splashing white again, toward the dark, the deep black and the occasional burst of light deep within the black, far away, weightless and silent, the distant, diamond-point explosions, among which she drifted slowly, wonderfully, in tears.

Alvin spoke to her about the Indians of Martha's Vineyard and how they had begun to press a claim for some lands at one end of the island, Gay Head, a place of moors and beaches, beach grass, low-lying bushes, dwarf trees hugging the dunes—no oil, so far as anyone knew—a few houses and a lighthouse, a barren place, it seemed to him, a place neither of crops nor livestock nor fishing harbors, a bleak place of back-yard vegetable gardens and wealthy stockbrokers, a place, perhaps, however, for a honeymoon when Kathy was well again and singing and he and she were married.

And she laughed, and alarmed herself with the dreadful
sound her laughter made.

She spat out the jello. She would not eat jello. It made her
sick. She spat it out. She kicked her leg. She pounded her fist.
Hurry up. How much? She kicked her leg.

Okay. Okay. No, no, no, no, no.

She grabbed Patrick by the arm.

How much?

How much what?

She scratched his arm. How much?

How much have you been through?

He told her of the operation, of how it had gone wrong, of
the catastrophe, of how everyone had thought that she was
dead, of how all this had been days ago, how this had been six
weeks ago, how she had revived and lapsed again, how she
had come in and out of consciousness, how she had kicked and
shaken her head, how everyone was doing all they could, how
terrible it had been, how horrible he had felt, how he had
cried, how he had prayed, how he had beat his fist against the
wall, how he had dreamed of her, how he had cried, how much
he loved her, how dreadful it had been, how unfair, how brutal
and how cruel, how no one could believe what had happened
to her, how no one knew what it had been, how the operation
was over now, and not much more could now be done.

And then she screamed, over and over—sounds, not
words—screamed loudly so that nurses came running to the
room, screamed over and over, sobbing screams, in waves and
spasms, and no one tried to stop her, but all stood silently and
watched.

Three

It was evident to Cunnought that she was no longer getting better. She recovered some functions and lost others, retrieved some new words, lost others, improved and deteriorated at the same time. Her condition was not stabilizing; she was collapsing into disorder again, dying again.

For several weeks, the nurses observed a range of symptoms that revealed no pattern. The patient fought and kicked; the patient was lethargic; the patient kicked and pulled at the ties that held her down. The patient was able to move her left extremities, understood but could not speak, banged the bed, shook her head, could not be roused, would neither eat nor drink, said yes or no to questions asked, opened eyes when spoken to but made no effort to reply, did not know her name, was difficult to rouse at night, would not eat nor drink, was heard to say, several times, "Oh, my God," and "somebody, please," had to have feeding tube placed in her throat in order to take nourishment, was heard to make noises as though choking, was heard to say, some time after the tube was removed,

"Oh, my God," did not speak, but seemed exceptionally alert.

Alvin explained to her that there was a reason for every-thing, that everything was explicable, and that, for the most part, everything was a matter of determination and will, that if one were tough and convinced and had faith and simply rea-soned one's way through a problem that there was no reason one could not come to a happy conclusion as, for instance, when he had once had a dream that his mother had been killed in an automobile accident, and so he had gotten in the car and driven to Tennessee to find her, and although she was not there when he arrived, he knew he could locate her if he just stayed with it and kept his determination, and, sure enough, he had found her at last with her sister in Kentucky and when he had walked in the door, she had just looked up and said very casually oh hi, Alvin—so, you see, nothing was wrong after all.

Besides, he said, I'll take care of you now.

No doctor or nurse had any hope that she would recover fully, and most of the more affectionate physicians thought that it would be very nice if she would die.

The staff blamed him, Cunnought believed, for what had happened to her; they blamed him and moved on, reckoning on her death, considering her a nuisance demanding of their time when other patients, patients who had some chance to recover, needed their care, patients who would reward their attention by living, patients who would not let them down. They left her with him, Cunnought believed, and did not wish him well. They hoped she died on him, in his presence, in his arms.

Some said that she was getting better. Alvin said she spoke more each day, that she moved her right arm and leg, that she understood more and more. Cunnought noted in the chart that

Alvin believed he had seen these phenomena, but Cunnought knew that she had not moved. Cunnought knew that much of the left parietal lobe had been wasted by the hemorrhage; the motor strip that controlled the right side of the body had been damaged or destroyed. She did not move that side of her body, no matter what Alvin thought he saw. Nor did she see him when he sat on the right side of her bed. Much of the occipital lobe of the left hemisphere had been destroyed; she was afflicted with a right homonomous hemianopsia; she saw nothing, from either eye, in her right field of vision. He could tell—on those occasions when she responded to something in her left field of vision, and saw nothing to her right.

Presumably, much of the language area near the left temporal lobe had been destroyed. She would not be able to read or write—certainly not well—if she recovered. Cunnought did not know whether she would ever be able to speak more than to say hurry up and please help and oh God.

He wondered how clearly she could think, whether the damage to her brain would alter the processes of her thought, whether the damage she had suffered meant she could no longer control her emotions quite as well, or understand the ones she felt, whether verbal and visual impressions would be so distorted as to be unpleasant, whether, indeed, the vision of a flower would cause such a degree of perceptual confusion as to be classifiable as pain.

It was possible that he would keep her alive only to discover that she would linger for twenty years or forty saying nothing, knowing nothing but confusion, helpless and deranged.

And yet he could not turn and run. Once a surgeon enters a patient, the patient belongs to him; they have wed one another; and he wished that he could understand himself then as the bridegroom whose acts of love would transform her, that he

could immerse himself in that consciousness that struggled and
subsided, rose to lucidity and ebbed, spoke and was silent,
whose urge to survive seemed not to be centered merely in a
will but rather in each neuron, each ion that collided, collapsed, rose in conflict, destroyed itself, collapsed, subsided.
He witnessed this, and, when some calamity seemed about to
overwhelm her, he joined in the struggle by assaulting the
body with antibiotics, or Mannitol, Decadron, Dilantin,
Phenobarbital. Then he would stand aside again and observe
the few signs that she gave of her enormous turmoil. He tried
to gaze at her steadily, without blinking, without pity, fear,
regret; he wished to consider her, as a guide in the wilderness
might regard his charges, with a bond even beyond love or
compassion.

He sat with her several times a day, first thing in the morning, during rounds in the afternoon, and at ten o'clock at night,
just before he went back home, across the bridge, to bed.

She watched him without blinking. He was crimson and
violent-eyed, shrieking with laughter, clad in a pale white
aura, with hands of burnt umber and holding in one hand a
curved sword of green jade and in the other a small brass bell,
in one hand a three-headed ax with incised blade and in the
other a yellow jonquil, in one hand a column of dancing fire
and in the other a lacquered cup of honey, in one hand a steel
dagger, glistening and needle-sharp and in the other a cool
stone, and he danced and whirled in front of her until his face
had no expression whatever, and he danced and whirled and
his scarves made the sound of the wind, and his head was
motionless and without expression, impassive as the stone,
fierce and gentle, terrible and lovely, and she embraced him
and drew him into her and danced with him.

He observed on a Wednesday, that her brain had begun to

swell again and push itself against the bandages at the site of the opening in her skull. He thought that the cerebrospinal fluid was not being properly absorbed back into her system, that it was building up pressure, causing the ventricles at the center of the brain to push out on the brain. What caused this swelling remained unknown. On Wednesday evening, he noted in the chart that the swelling persisted.

On Thursday morning, the patient was taken down to the radiology laboratory for X-ray pictures of her head, and it appeared that the ventricles might be somewhat enlarged. The brain had begun to swell again—not for the same reason that it had swelled in the operating room; this time it swelled more slowly. Cunnought asked several other physicians to look at the X-rays, and the others could not agree that the ventricles were so distended as to suggest hydrocephalus. Swollen perhaps, but not enough to suggest that they were the cause of the patient's deteriorating condition. She was dying once again, and once again, no one knew quite why.

He commenced, then, to perform spinal taps—inserting long, flexible needles into her spine and draining out a quantity of spinal fluid, to reduce the total amount of cerebrospinal fluid in the spine and brain, to shrink the ventricles and so to relieve the pressure that enlarged the ventricles and pushed out against the brain.

After he performed the spinal tap, he sat with her for a while to see whether he might sense any change in symptoms. Not long before, Cunnought had reported at a conference of neurosurgeons on a case that had gone wrong. He had removed an entire vertebra from the spine of a middle-aged man, and eventually the man completely recovered. But, in the course of the operation, he encountered massive bleeding, and altogether the man had to be given twenty-four units of blood by transfusion—twice the number of units an adult male ordinarily has in his system. Well, one of the neurosurgeons from Sweden said, I want you to know that we performed three identical operations and made the same mistake in each one, as we mentioned in our paper (implying that Cunnought had not kept up with the Swedish literature) before we changed our approach.

So Cunnought told his friend Henry of Kathy Morris. Henry was horrified; he had never heard of such a case. Told of the slow swelling that occurred in the weeks after the operation, the lack of clear symptoms of hydrocephalus, Henry had no idea what Cunnought should do.

She had not improved by the following day, and, once again, Cunnought performed a spinal tap and sat for a while at her bedside. He wished to see a change in symptoms, but he could not say certainly that she had improved. Lift your left hand, he said, but she did not move. Open your eyes, Kathy, he said, it's Dr. Cunnought. Kathy, how are you? When he pinched her, she still did not move, and so he clenched his fist, and, with his knuckles, bore in harshly in the middle of her chest, and then she groaned.

By the next day, she had not yet improved. He performed another spinal tap.

He sent her to the radiology laboratory for another X-ray study. Still he could not declare with any confidence that the ventricles were swollen. No other physician would reassure him on the point. None believed she had hydrocephalus. Cunnought believed he might take her back into the operating room and install a shunt—a tube that pierces directly through the brain and down into the ventricles to drain the spinal fluid. A shunt, once placed into the ventricular system, remains there, a permanent piece of equipment. The external end of the tube is connected to the patient's circulatory system at a point in the neck, and so the spinal fluid is drained back down into the patient's blood supply. The tiny tube that performs this feat is buried neatly under the scalp and the flesh of the neck and cannot be seen by any casual observer. The principle of the operation is simple enough, and yet the risks are ever-present: the tube is sent down through the frontal lobe of the cortex—damaging the least understood area of the brain; and, if the surgeon misses the ventricles on his first pass, he must retreat and plunge in again and again. If the ventricles are greatly swollen, they are easy to hit. If not, as in Kathy's case, the surgeon may have to make repeated attempts. And Cunnought could find no one who thought the operation was called for. No one detected symptoms that pointed clearly to hydro-cephalus. Cunnought considered the prospects of certain damage to the brain—a brain that could hardly tolerate more damage—against the remote chance that the procedure would be at all useful.

If she had hydrocephalus, a spinal tap should relieve pressure and so she ought to recover somewhat, temporarily. Temporary recovery would indicate correct diagnosis. Temporary recovery would indicate that a shunt was called for. And yet, it seemed to Cunnought, though he looked for symptoms of improvement, though he sometimes imagined that he saw such symptoms, in fact she was getting steadily worse, and that the spinal taps made no difference whatever.

At a cocktail party at the Rockefeller University, Cunnought circulated cheerily among the surgeons from Bellevue and St. Barnabas, drinking Scotch, mentioning mutual friends, working in a reference to an interesting case, young woman, meningioma, massive swelling (what?) during the operation (no idea, never heard), subsequent slow swelling, as though it were hydrocephalus but without the swollen ventricles—utter mystery, no idea, never heard of such a thing. He wandered among his peers, like a stockbroker at a Westport cocktail party seeking free medical opinions. He gleaned from the assembled guests the reports—none of them firsthand—of three similar cases of inexplicable swelling of the brain during an operation. The essential difference between these cases and that of Kathy Morris was that none of these other three patients left the operating room alive.

Cunnought returned to the hospital after his party at The Rockefeller University, and he sat by Kathy's bedside and administered yet another spinal tap. She did not respond at all. No surgery was called for. He sat with her a while longer, and, as he sat with her, he reasoned that there was nothing else that he could do—he knew of nothing else to try but this surgery—and, with this operation, she would either recover or die.

Four

Dr. Palamara wheeled her into the operating room that day, a fine, sunny morning, April now, and the light, reflected from the Cathedral, suffused the room, and seemed to bring the outdoors in. Palamara completed the small burr hole in the top of the skull, and then, through that, Cunnought placed the long, slender tube into the ventricle.

Anne, pretty, brown-haired, slender single woman with angular features and brown eyes, directly focused, alert and calm, wearing Pucci underclothes, recalled the man who loved her, to whom she was to be married, who married another young woman (a girl then) asking Anne whether she thought it would be romantic for him to fly his own plane with his new bride to a honeymoon in Canada. No, she said, not on your honeymoon. Be superstitious just this once: never trust a newlywed to fly his own small plane. Rule of thumb. I don't know where I am, he broadcast on his radio from somewhere on the Canadian border; I'm emptying the gas tanks and going down.

Cunnought placed the tube quickly, deftly, casually it seemed, and—on the first attempt—perfectly.

Palamara closed—with a meticulous stitch, an inconspicuously cosmetic stitch that would be unnoticeable to most of the patient's friends in the event she survived.

Five

The patient was awake and alert by six o'clock in the evening, still awake and alert two hours later, and later still the patient was awake and alert. The patient looked at the examiner very intently, and the examiner asked another nurse to come to the bedside. The patient was awake and alert and able to move her right arm for the first time in more than a month.

The next morning, the patient awoke crying like a small child.

Patrick arrived at the hospital and thought that she looked as though she had just awakened from a long sleep. She smiled at him and cried and looked around the room, smiling and crying. Patrick thought that she cried just the way he remembered that their mother cried. Her first words, which she repeated over and over as she cried, were: This boy loves his mother.

PART FOUR

One

I am Kathy Morris, she said, when Cunnought came in the door that first morning after the operation. I am Kathy Morris. He thought he might fall down, and so, he stood still for several moments to make certain his gait was steady. She spoke again: I am Kathy Morris.

He went to her bedside then and asked her to move her right arm, which she did, and then her right leg, which she did. She could still not see anything in her right field of vision—and Cunnought knew that she would never be able to see to her right side. Who am I? Cunnought asked her, and she said nothing. Am I your doctor?—and she nodded yes.

Who is this?

She said nothing.

Is this your brother?

She nodded.

Are you in church?

She shook her head.

Are you in a hospital?

She nodded.

What am I holding? Is this a glass of water?

She nodded.

Is this a water pitcher?

She nodded.

What have you just been doing? Have you been skiing?

She shook her head.

Have you just had an operation?

She nodded.

How are you? Are you going to be okay now?

She neither nodded nor shook her head. She looked fiercely at Cunnought.

You are going to be okay now.

She lay quietly for a day, saying nothing, but responding to all requests of doctors and nurses. Gradually, it occurred to her that her room was empty. For a long time, it was dark, and she heard no sound; she was alone. She felt perfectly clear-headed and even elated. She was aware of the silence, of the scent of disinfectant in the air, of the coldness of the steel bars on the sides of her bed—all sensations that she had not noticed before.

But she was still not entirely, reliably sure whether she was alive or dead. She decided she needed to get out of the hospital, and she was found half an hour later, by one of the nurses, dangling over the side bars of her bed, held there by the ties on her arms and legs, smiling.

The nurse called in a commotion of interns and other nurses, and they put her back in bed.

After they left, she called out: hello, hello there! and, when a nurse came back into the room, she smiled at the nurse. When the nurse left, she called out again, hello there! hello there! and smiled once again when the nurse returned. The nurse promised a cup of coffee if she would be quiet, and she helped Kathy drink the coffee. When she was finished, Kathy said hello and smiled. Hello, Kathy said again, hello, hello. And the nurse said hello.

She practiced saying her name over and over again, accenting first one syllable, then another, and, when the nurse said my name is Mary Anne, Kathy repeated that name again and again, and then when the nurse said coffee she said coffee, and then the word cup, coffee I forget, coffee cup, cup on the table, bed, Kathy in the bed. My name is Kathy Morris, coffee in the cup I'm on the I forget, bed, Mary Anne. Hello. I am Kathy Morris in a bed on the I forget in a room, how are you I am fine, thank you very much, thank you very much (she took Mary Anne's hand and rubbed it against her cheek) thank you very much.

The next day, Cunnought observed that she was able to move both her right arm and leg easily. She said hello when he entered the room, but she declined otherwise to speak to him. She turned her back to him.

Well, Cunnought said, I know you're mad at me, but I thought you were going to sing for me when your operation was finished.

She turned to look at him.

Aren't you going to sing for me?

Sing?

Why don't you sing "Happy Birthday"?

Sing?

Sure.

Happy birthday to you . . .

Not bad. How about row your boat.

Row, row, row your boat . . . (She commenced to cry.)

Not bad. What else do you know? Do you know "I Left My Heart in San Francisco"?

I left my heart in San Francisco . . . (She cried.)

I don't suppose you know any old Beatles songs?

I used to know my I forget my favorite one.

What was that?

There are places I remember

in my life (she cried)

though some have changed . . .

some are gone . . .

all these places

have their meanings . . . I can sing.

Yes.

Did you hear me? I can sing?

Yes.

Is it a miracle?

Yes.

I'm not a bad singer, am I?

You're a great singer.

Oh, God, I can sing.

Cunnought wrote in her chart (smugly): Beginning to sing (altho off key).

By the time Patrick arrived, she was sitting up in bed. Her fingernails were painted a dazzling shade of red from a bottle of polish given her by one of the nurses; she wore brilliant red lipstick; and she was eating a pint of Rocky Road ice cream. This is mine, she said to Patrick, you can't have it. You can eat ice cream, he said. I can sing, too, she said. Can you sing "Happy Birthday"? No, I can sing I left my heart in San Francisco, raindrops keep falling. I can sing anything, Patrick, I didn't mean to cry, but that's what I do now, I sing and cry and sing and cry, that's what I can do, oh I have a wonderful time, every day I have a wonderful time, I'm having a lovely day, I love every time I have, would you like to hear me sing?

M-I-C-K-E-Y M-O-U-S-E
Mickey Mouse, da-da-da-da
Mickey Mouse, da-da-da-da
Do you want some ice cream?

Doctor Palamara and the others from the recovery room, the residents and anesthesiologists, nurses from the operating service, radiologists, orderlies who had pushed her cart, people from the social services department reported first to her room to say to her, gee, you sure gave us a scare, and then, afterward, went to their jobs. Everyone wanted to see her perform her new feats.

She discovered that she wished to try things.

> Patient continues to improve. Vital signs stable. Patient able to eat with chopsticks.

The nurses helped her to walk; her name was written on a piece of paper for her, and she traced it over and over; she said that, although she had difficulty speaking, she was able to think of the words even if she could not say them aloud; she was concerned about her appearance and wished to wear a scarf over her head; on occasion she would have difficulty remembering people's names; she was helped to walk; she was able to eat her meals by herself; she was eager to help the nurses help her; she was able to walk on her own with a walker; she seemed increasingly aware of her surroundings, able to remember some events of the past, but still had difficulty in speaking of them, was able to walk to her physical therapy by herself.

Some tricks still eluded her. Asked to close her eyes, she could not identify a coin when it was placed in her right hand. When a pen was placed in her right hand, she would turn it over and over in her hand, feeling it, gripping it, saying oh, yes, oh, yes—unable to name it. She could not feel heat or cold on her right side. She could not see to the right. Both sensory and visual areas of the left hemisphere had been damaged.

Thus, she could not play the piano, because she could not feel her right hand on the keyboard. She would not be able to dance in a musical comedy or move dexterously about the stage in an opera, because she could not see to her right, could not sense her position on stage.

Even worse, when asked to pretend to kick a football with her left foot, she would sit immobile, bewildered. She could visualize the act at once; but the three-part instruction was too complex for her to carry out. She would kick with her right foot, or touch her left leg, or try to repeat the instruction and fail even at that. When asked to shoot a gun with her right hand, she would smile and shoot with her left hand.

She could not translate a visual image—an image that sprang to her mind at once—into language or into expressive action.

Even if she might learn to compensate for her blindness and lack of sensation on her right side, what would she do if a theatrical director were to tell her to dance three steps to the right and kick, to turn upstage and wave goodbye with her right hand, to waltz downstage left and kiss the leading man?

Patrick had brought her guitar to the hospital, and she held it comfortably, and moved the fingers of her left hand nimbly over the strings. But she could not pluck the strings with the fingers of her right hand without giving the matter such prolonged and particular attention as to make the maneuver into a metaphysical ordeal.

Still, she could sing in nightclubs. She could stand, without moving, and sing in nightclubs. She could hold the microphone, or keep her hands at her sides, or hold the microphone with her right hand and gesture with her left. She could look to both sides of the stage. She could move her right side, after all; her right side was perfectly strong. She could stand on one leg and then another with her eyes closed. She could hop up and down on one foot and then hop up and down on the other. She could walk. She could stand and walk without tottering or falling. She could mount a stage. She could stand and sing in front of a microphone. She would sing thus. Judy Collins, she seemed to remember, had been through a great deal. Judy Collins was blonde and large-boned, a grown woman, mature, not a child, not a girl, a mother in fact, a grown mature woman who understood the ways of luck and such, in short a woman. She neither danced, nor played the piano, nor played the guitar, at least not always.

When Kathy had been six years old, her mother had dressed her up in silly childish dresses, crinolines, godknows whatall silly puffed out dresses, and she sang "Puff the Magic Dragon," and her mother played the piano while she sang, and while she sings now, often, she can hear her mother playing still. She would sing she thought she could not do otherwise.

Cunnought was concerned only that Kathy no longer showed any special energy. Even people who have attempted suicide are elated after they have been rescued. But she was tranquil, as though she had spent her will and had none left. She was disturbingly peaceful and carefree. He wished she would show some sign of that euphoric flight into health that invariably foreshadowed recovery.

Cunnought asked a friend, a neurologist, to examine her. Brust, the friend, was a young man, no more than forty, cordial but aloof, attentive and impassive. He was a student and collector of Japanese art, a connoisseur of Japanese movies, an omnivorous reader—whose tastes ran to the more complex novels, to Pynchon, Barth, Barthelme, and Gaddis—and he had made a personal specialty of studying language.

He sat bolt upright and was precise in manner—a logician who believed that the instruments of reason were manifestly more exact than knives in dissecting the mysteries of the brain.

He believed that the musician—and painter, and the mathematician, and the poet—wielded a better scalpel than the surgeon when it came to limning the structures and traceries of the brain in all their delicacy and tact and discretion. He examined her with sentences and words; he sent propositions down deep within her brain to see what might be returned to him; and he probed the order and ruin of her brain by driving a line of clarity and simplicity into her mind to observe how it was blurred or distorted or broken. He betrayed the same highstrung alertness that Cunnought showed in the operating room, and, as he spoke and listened, he wrote constantly, with barely perceptible movements of his fingers, in the air.

He showed her, first, a chart on which six letters were printed and asked her to point to the *L,* and then to the *H*. She hesitated for a painfully long time before she found both letters. He asked her then to point out the geometrical shapes on another chart as he named them: a circle, a square, a triangle, a spiral. She had to guess at the triangle and the spiral.

Asked to identify the pictures showing people smoking, drinking, sleeping, she was fast and certain. She was sure of most colors—blue, pink, gray, red—and could identify numbers by counting silently up to them—and guessing at the larger ones such as *70* and *700*.

She could point, on request, to her nose, her ear, her shoulder, but not her ankle. She could not find her middle finger and she required several minutes of silent thought each time she needed to distinguish left from right.

What's this?

Oh, yes, that's your . . . I don't know. Can you tell me?

Elbow.

Your elbow.

(Pointing to his wrist.) What's this?

Your pulse.

What is it?

Your pulse.

I had in mind the word *wrist*.

Yes, wrist.

Will a board sink in water?

No.

Will a stone sink in water?

Yes.

Is a hammer good for cutting wood?

(Silence.)

No.

Do two pounds of flour weigh more than one?

No.

Is one pound of flour heavier than two?

Would you say that again?

Is one pound of flour heavier than two?

Yes.

Can you tell me the days of the week?

Monday. Tuesday. Wednesday. Did I say Tuesday?

Yes.

Tuesday. Wednesday. Saturday.

Can you tell me the months of the year?

Yes. January. February. January. February. March. January. It's just the first couple months that I forget.

Now if you will just repeat these words after me: *chair*.

Chair.

Circle.

Circle.

Fifteen.

Fifteen.

Hammock.

Ham . . . ham . . . ock.

Triangle.

Tri . . . ang . . . angle . . .

Dripping.

Drizzle.

Brown.

Brown.

Methodist.

Protestant.

What?

I just wondered if you were paying attention.

Methodist.

Metho . . . meth . . . dister . . . meth . . . o . . . dist . . .

Now I want you to think of some names of things for me.
What do we tell time with?

A watch.

What do you do with a razor?

Shave.

What do we cut paper with?

A knife—or, you know, or with scissors.

What color is grass?

Brown?

What color is coal?

Black.

How many things in a dozen?

Ten?

How many animals in the zoo can you name?

Okay. Monkeys (silence), zebras (silence), tigers, bears, lions.

(Silence.)

Bears. Did I tell you that?

Yes.

(Silence.)

Now I want you to read the short sentences on this page:

YOU KNOW HOW.

You know me.

DOWN TO EARTH.

Down in earth.

I GOT HOME FROM WORK.

I got home before work. I got home for . . . no . . .

THEY HEARD HIM SPEAK ON THE RADIO LAST NIGHT.

Something about a radio last night.

THE BARN SWALLOW CAPTURED A PLUMP WORM.

The barn swallowing . . . a capitol or something . . . this is a worm.

THE LAWYER'S CLOSING ARGUMENT CONVINCED HIM.

The lawyer lost . . . no . . . something about a case . . .

Cunnought was depressed, and Brust, although he labored to maintain his formal demeanor, was both dejected by her showing and impressed by her persistence. Kathy alone

showed neither fatigue nor unhappiness but recovered her
energy after each small defeat and pressed on to the next
question.

Now I am going to spell out some words aloud, and I want
you to tell me what they are.

N-O.

No.

M-A-N.

Man.

G-I-R-L.

Is that a girl?

W-H-I-P.

Milk.

B-L-A-C-K.

Again please?

B-L-A-C-K.

Bark?

E-L-B-O-W.

I don't know that one.

W-H-I-S-K-E-Y.

I can't say that.

Now would you write the words as I speak them: SOFT.

No, I can't write that.

S-O-F-T.

Thank you.

BELONG.

I'm sorry, I can't write that.

B-E-L-O-N-G.

No, I'm sorry. I still can't.

Would you write your name and address for me?

She wrote her name very slowly and meticulously, and just
the first few characters of her address and then he stopped her

and asked her very quietly if she would copy some few sentences he would write. She could not do that, and so he told
her—his voice still exceedingly quiet—that the last task he
would give her was to ask her to write the proper identifying
words under several pictures.

For key, she wrote K-E.

For fifteen, she wrote F-I.

For red, she wrote R-E.

And for circle, she wrote A.

He put his hand on hers then and said, good, that's fine.
You've done enough now.

They sat silently for a while, and she asked, at last, how am
I?

And Brust said, I think you're going to do very well indeed.

Yes, thank you, but I want to know exactly how I am. Why
am I going to do well?

Because you are very intelligent and extremely determined.

Would you tell me more please?

Okay. You have sustained extensive damage to the left
hemisphere of your brain. You are aphasic, which means you
have trouble with the comprehension and use of language.
There are many forms of aphasia: Wernicke's aphasia, which
involves difficulty in naming or repeating words and is usually
associated with damage to the left temporal lobe. Then there
are lesions in the inferior frontal lobe—in Broca's area. . . .
But, none of this is of any use to you. In fact, you have some
symptoms of many different syndromes. Agraphia, acalculia,
right-left confusion, and finger agnosia are generally accounted the signs of Gerstmann's syndrome. Is knowing that
of any use to you? Do you understand what I'm telling you?

I understand you perfectly. Which of these do I have?

You appear to fit in a group, having a very rare syndrome,

identified by Geschwind, the isolation of the speech area; but all this is extremely tentative and arbitrary. It may well be that all classifications are wrong. There may be a virtually infinite number of aphasias. I'm inclined to think so. Some things do not have just one explanation, or interpretation, or cause. Some things are unnameable.

Yes, I know that.

Language is not speech, or reading, or writing. It is the making of propositions about the world. The making of propositions about the world does not depend on this neuron or that, this area of the brain or that, the memory of this word or ability to construct that phrase, it depends upon the whole of your consciousness. And I am not able to tell you anything important about that. I can only tell you that I am astonished that you and I can speak with one another.

Am I going to get better?

I don't know. You'll see.

Why can I sing?

It may be one of your few pieces of luck. The lyrics to songs are not only bits of language but, because you sing them, they are also bits of music. As such, they appear to be stored in your right hemisphere, too. Perhaps not entirely, but at least enough to give you the boost you need. Do you have a hard time starting to sing, thinking of the first few words before you begin to sing?

Yes.

And then, once you start to sing, once the words become music as it were, then you remember them without trouble.

Yes. Can I learn new songs?

Can you?

Yes. Is that a miracle? I know it's amazing, but is it a

miracle that I go through all this and music comes out? I mean, if there is such a thing, then this must be a miracle, right?

What kind of songs do you sing?

Oh, I have some new songs to write about, where I've been, what I've seen, you know, the usual things: yellow birds, the sounds of daffodils, notes of pastel blue.

Of course.

All that stood in the way of going on with her career was the fact that, when Cunnought had noticed that the brain was swelling in the midst of the operation, and he had had to step back from the table to see whether he could do anything to control the swelling and bleeding, he had stopped in midoperation. He had not—he had neglected to tell her this—removed all of the tumor.

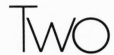

Two

He told her at last one day: he said that she would need to
return to the operating room to have an acrylic plate fitted to
her skull—the left hemisphere of her brain was still protected
only by a layer of muscle and scalp—and that, at the same
time, he would need just to have a look to see whether the
tumor was entirely removed.

You mean I still have a tumor in my head? When you had to
stop, you had to leave part of the tumor there.

Yes.

How big is it?

About the size of a walnut.

Oh God, I'm not sure I can handle this.

I think you can.

I don't think I can go through it all again. What can happen
now?

Anything.

All over again.

Yes.

200

Oh, boy.

She was dizzy when he left that day, and she thought she might not have the rest of the tumor removed, that she might just live with it for a while, have a career, however long or short, and then just die. On the other hand, she thought she might go to another surgeon, a more fatherly sort of man, someone gentler, less cocky, less ready to plunge ahead, someone just slightly less eager to get into the operating room, someone who did not quite like to perform surgery. She wanted to run, she wanted to get drunk or stoned, and yet she could not run from dread or terror as her father had done, she could not run from the prospect of loneliness or disaster or confusion, she must return and face him with his jade sword and silk scarves, and then, too, she discovered that she trusted him.

Three

She thought that it was too beautiful a day to die, and, as she was wheeled into the operating room and saw the familiar overhead light, the view of the Cathedral, Tsing and Anne, she wished that she could stay awake, for it seemed absurd to be asleep for the best part.

She dozed and Cunnought roused her, and she said oh, how are you?

Fine.

I remember you.

That's a good sign.

I feel as though we're going dancing.

The anesthesiologists moved in on her then, with intravenous lines and monitors, and just before she went to sleep she said I'm very cold.

It was possible to see out, beyond the Cathedral, all the way to Central Park. It was a clear, brisk day, and the physicians and nurses in the operating room savored it and took their time preparing for the surgery. Cunnought had wanted the same people who had been with him for the first operation to assist at this one—to make him feel comfortable, and to see it go well this time. The resident was different—Luddy had gone on to another service, and his place was taken by Celia.

Cunnought took his time arranging the X-rays on the light box, adjusting the overhead light, checking the strap on his magnifying glasses. A microscope, mounted on a mobile stand, had been placed in a corner of the operating room. No exceptionally fine work would be performed in this operation, and the presence of the microscope in the room was outlandish.

Celia was intrigued by the scope, and asked Cunnought if he were having trouble finding his way across the room to the operating table.

What's that?

You can always tell when a surgeon's over the hill; he needs the scope to see. I thought you said you were only thirty-five.

Yeah.

If I used a scope everyone would say it's just because I'm a woman.

And we all know that's not true, right, Celia?

Celia watched then as Cunnought moved the operating table first one way and then another, adjusting it minutely, changing its position by a mere inch or two forward and back, and then Celia became somewhat quieter, recognizing that he was procrastinating before going back into this familiar skull and its freshly remembered catastrophes, that he needed to perform certain ritual acts to invite the favor of the gods.

Then he had shaved her head, and he had no excuse left not to start. The incision would begin in the scalp that covered the skull high up toward the midline, and then the knife would have to come down directly over brain, where no protective bone remained. Before, when Cunnought had finally closed the wound, before he had grafted facialata—a sheath of gristly muscle from the thigh—over the opening in the cranium. The facialata took the place of dura and so, for this operation, he would cut down through scalp, a layer of muscle—no bone—and through the facialata to the brain.

Because he cut through scar tissue, the blood flowed especially freely, and although he was not concerned, because he knew the reason for the bleeding, he moved swiftly to stanch the flow.

On his honeymoon in the Bahamas, he and Janet went snorkeling for the first time off Nassau. Out in a boat in shark-infested waters, one of their party surfaced, calling out: tiger shark. Cunnought was on the boat. Another man, standing with him, asked: are you coming—and the other man dove in. Cunnought dove at once, terrified; and then, as soon as he got his head underneath the surface where he could see what was happening, he wasn't scared at all.

To make certain that an incision in the scalp would not penetrate facialata and brain, Cunnought announced to his assistants that he would use blunt dissection to separate scalp from facia, and, with that, he slipped his fingers in an opening between scalp and facia and pulled upward—tearing and clawing, ripping the flesh from the head it seemed—pulling the scalp up and away from the brain.

Then, having come upon the facialata, he employed that most elegant of surgical maneuvers: he flicked a small incision in the facia; inserted the Freer elevator; placed the knife lightly on the flat face of the elevator; and skimmed along the facia, protecting the brain with the face of the elevator, cutting open the facia with the blade of the knife.

You're laying on the Decadron, are you?

Yes, doctor.

Decadron inhibits brain swelling, sometimes. No one knows how it works, when it does. Cunnought ordered the maximum dose. It was, he said, like saying a prayer.

Oh, God, he said.

Is that good god or bad god, Celia asked.

Just oh, God, this brain is bad, this brain absolutely lacks any architecture at all.

Everyone was silent as Cunnought went down into the brain. It seemed to Celia that he was disoriented, and unable now to find the tumor. Nothing appeared to be precisely in its proper place in this ravaged brain, and Cunnought proceeded to search for the tumor with excruciating slowness. He seemed to Celia to be profoundly unhappy.

He wished Jean Shepherd were with him then. He thought Shepherd must be a very lonely guy, talking through the night on his radio show and hearing no one answer him.

There it is, he said. I think that's it, but it really looks too small.

Is that it?

It looks awfully small. It looks like dura.

What?

No, it can't be dura.

Is that the tumor?

That looks like tumor, but no, that has a big vein going through it. That can't be it. This brain is really terrible. Oh God, that's it, that's it, there it is.

He was convinced instantly that she was going to die.

I'll tell you what, he said at last, let's just leave it alone. We won't take it out now, we'll just leave it there.

No one replied to him.

Four

He scouted the entire periphery of the tumor, then, looking for tiny blood vessels, cauterizing them all meticulously, obsessively, moving around and around the tumor, laying the tumor bare, and creating an utterly bloodless field. He stood back for several minutes and watched, to make certain no drop of blood appeared anywhere. Then, Cunnought turned to Celia and asked her to remove the tumor.

She took it neatly, with several cautious but exact passes of the knife, and then she, too, cauterized—closing the few remaining minute vessels that had been just beneath the tumor. They both stood for several minutes, watching for any trace of blood, and, finding none, Cunnought took a syringe filled with sterile water and flushed the area of the operation again and again and again, saying that the water must run until it is as clear as a mountain stream, and then, looking one last time for several minutes, he declared that they were ready to close.

He placed the hard acrylic plate carefully, edge to edge with the opening in the skull, overlapping somewhat to hold it in its place, and stitched it in, drew the muscle and the scalp over it and closed slowly and with care.

Five

He took his time, nipping away the stitches that held the sterile drapes around her head, clearing away the overhead table of instruments, taking the sterile drapes in his right hand and sweeping them away to the floor, saying quietly, involuntarily under his breath as he saw her face—eyes closed and damp, her neck, bare shoulders and torso—Helloooo, Kathy.

He moved around beside her, then, and took the tape from her eyelids and gently lifted her head and wrapped it in the large, white turban of bandages, carefully, leisurely.

Do they teach you that in neurosurgery school, Celia asked.

What's that?

To take so long with the bandages you'll never know whether she wakes up or not?

I am finished, said Cunnought. You can wake her up now.

Tsing gave her the intravenous antidotes to her anesthesia and curare and then Cunnought put his hand gently on her shoulder and said, Okay, Kathy, open your eyes.

She was silent and did not move. Cunnought did not speak again for several moments.

All right, Kathy, you may wake up now, your operation is over, and you're fine.

She opened up her eyes.

I'm alive?

Yes, you're alive.

Oh, God.

She reached out to take Cunnought's hand.

I'm very cold.

You'll be warm in just a moment.

I can speak.

Yes.

She reached up and touched his cheek and held him, her hand on the side of his head.

Oh, hey, she said, thank you.

Six

Cunnought wished she would show some interest in working on her music again. She spoke of what she might do, but she did nothing; her passivity had begun to cause him ever-present anxiety. Perhaps her visions of singing had become more pleasurable than singing itself; perhaps her dreams had become sufficient for her.

Alvin thought that she was a bit slower to smile, somewhat simplified somehow, and somehow younger. He felt, too, that she was leaving him, moving on, drifting away from him. He hated, in truth, to see her get better. Now that she had made it, he thought, she had abandoned him; she was, for him, dead. He told her that he could not believe she could feel nothing on her right side, that she must feel something there, that anyone could see her right side was perfectly okay and perhaps the nerves there only needed to be awakened after the operation, stimulated back into functioning. He believed that to be the case, he told her, and so—for a time, as long as she would allow him—he came to the hospital every day and pinched her

right side, her arm, leg, foot, hip, kidneys, pinched and hit
her, pummeled her, rabbit-punched her, worked his knuckles
into her side, grasped her flesh and tugged and wrenched and
twisted, until at last, she told him that was enough, and he
stopped coming.

Jay thought that she was, on the whole, calmer than he had
known her to be for a long time, perhaps calmer than he had
ever known her to be. She seemed less hip, less sure of herself,
more mature. She seemed more aware of others. He thought
she had become a woman.

Still, Cunnought observed, she was entirely passive, and he
commenced to become alarmed about it. She dozed and day-
dreamed, considering, half-awake, the first lesson Miss
Bampton would give her at the music school, in the Toscanini
Room there, with the deep, soft easychairs, flower-patterned
slip covers, golden carpet, Renaissance cabinet, bust (of
whom?), Venetian blinds, incongruous fluorescent ceiling
fixtures and green walls reminiscent of the hospital, and how,
out of the disaster area of her head, bombed out, shattered
ruins, splayed and benumbed, rubble of a head, shards, fragments, broken images, statues, pieces of colonnade, half-lost
inscription, smashed phrases, letters and numerals, fragments
of a lost age, strewn and now to be regathered, bits piled up on
top of one another, new walls, arches, buttresses, half-
forgotten romanesque, flying buttress, stained glass window,
new light, lift, incandescence, song, air, variation, she would
sing: Se mia speranza, se mia joia, se mia bene, se mia pace,
se mia speranza—short of breath, she would have to recon-
struct the old songs—an easy chore, she now knew—and fling
the new songs back in among the bits of rubble, make them old
somehow so that she could recall them, incorporate them
somehow amid wreckage so that she could dance lightly over

the past with her notes and pluck the words with the notes, lightly, pluck the words with wings of notes attached, give them flight, stay loose, open up, depend less upon the old structures, no longer so dependable, trust the intricacies, complexities, curiosities, amazingness, wonderfulness, possibility of the new disaster area. To make music of this, surely, would be a miracle, which she realized she could perform with ease.

She did not wish to complain, but she could not help noticing that her visitors had stopped coming to see her. She wondered what had happened to them. They might be tired, of course. Now that she was alive, they might need a vacation themselves. No doubt they were tired. Perhaps, too, they were bored with her. Perhaps, indeed, they were bored because they sensed, now that she was alive, she would not improve any more.

Or perhaps, she considered with a sudden start, they were there, but she was dozing off again, drifting unconscious again without realizing it. Perhaps these periods of lucidity were only momentary. Perhaps she was still not entirely conscious, entirely intact, alive. Perhaps most pieces were missing from her life and she did not realize it because she was still in the artificial world of the hospital. Perhaps if she tried to go out into the streets she would realize that entire swatches of life were invisible to her. Perhaps, just as she could not see to her right, so she would not be able to experience entire chunks of life, whole neighborhoods, days, meals, weeks at a time. Perhaps she was not alive after all; perhaps she was a vegetable, destined to remain forever in the hospital, smiling, eating breakfast, sitting, staring, whole afternoons vanishing. She thought she would not know unless she could see all of it, touch it, sit in it, or whether she would only be able to remember part of it.

On the way back from her physical therapy class one day, she walked out the front door of the hospital.

She had on blue jeans, a football jersey, and fluffy blue slippers and her head was swathed in silk scarves, and she thought she looked mad, but then, she reckoned, New York's streets are full of crazy-looking people.

She was spotted at the corner by one of the orderlies, Felix, who asked her where she was going.

I can't talk to you now. I have to go.

What do you mean you have to go?

I have to go. I'll tell you what. You come with me.

They set off along 110th Street, heading for her old apartment near the music school, and the world looked real to her, and she thought she was alive and sane and somewhat intact as they made their way up Broadway past the pushers and flaked-out drunks, the corner preacher handing out leaflets, newsdealer, purveyor of stolen wristwatches, and she was overcome with a sudden longing for the world, a sudden terrific physical love of colors and sounds and of the acrid and too-sweet odors of the street, and of the sensation of her feet upon the sidewalk. She pointed out to Felix the dark greens and the light, the silver green and the citrine.

The alarm went out among the nurses, doctors, administrators, hospital guards at the doors, that she had escaped. They called the police. They sent search parties out into the streets around the neighborhood. They called her brother, phoned her uncle, her friends Alvin, Jay, Liz. At last, in desperation, and in fear of what he might say, one of the residents telephoned to Dr. Cunnought and told him of the disaster and asked him what to do.

Oh, that's absolutely great, he said. Now, just let her go.

Afterword

Several months ago, Dr. Brust examined Kathy Morris once again and found that her speech had improved to such an extent—her intelligence was so keen, and her ability to get around any frustrations so adept—that no one would notice in casual conversation that she had any difficulty at all. She still missed an occasional word, but she divined the gist of another's remarks quickly, and, in her reply, made sure she covered any question by surrounding the topic of conversation—by saying more than she perhaps needed to say, watching her fellow conversationalist closely for clues to where she might have gone astray, where she was secure, navigating the shoals of conversation deftly, with swift, light, corrective strokes, a jest, a smile. She seemed sometimes to talk her way around a subject with bright, improvisational chatter, running off in tangents and coming back to the main theme, not merely free-associating but leaping to new themes, too, like a jazz player. She seemed loquacious at times—but when she sensed her talk running away with her, she would catch herself up and say cheerily, Well, you tell me, or I give up, or You guess, I don't know.

All these stratagems would be accounted merely mannerisms—attractive, and sometimes flirtatious—by a stranger. No one meeting her for the first time now would notice anything extraordinary about her. Her hair is still short, but fashionably so. She seems somewhat hesitant at times. She tends to wish to have people stand or walk to her left, or, at lunch, to take the chair to the left. She still cannot see to her right, and so she cannot safely drive a car. She cannot play the piano. She cannot play classical guitar; her sense of "place" in her right hand is not good enough to pluck the strings; but she can strum the guitar. She cannot read or write—either words or music—on a level much better than that of a third grade student; but her reading and writing, both of words and music, show some promise of slow improvement.

She is able to sing. She can sing anything, both new songs and old. She learns her songs by listening to them over and over again, and she knows them thoroughly this way. Her other musical abilities are utterly intact: she has a perfect sense of rhythm, pitch, tone, attack. She is now, once again, at the beginning of her career as a singer.

I saw her not long ago at a suburban nightclub just outside New York City, a small place with something of the feeling of a neighborhood pub, densely populated by a young crowd, and with a small stage at the far end of the room, lit with three or four baby spots. She did a set with a piano player, bass, and drummer. She began quietly, and at first the music contended with the sounds of murmuring voices, the snap of cigarette lighters, the sharp riff of ice cubes. But as she went on there were no sounds but the music, the audience was absolutely silent, she was in command, and then she sang flat-out and terrifically, and with amazing passion.